the exercisebible

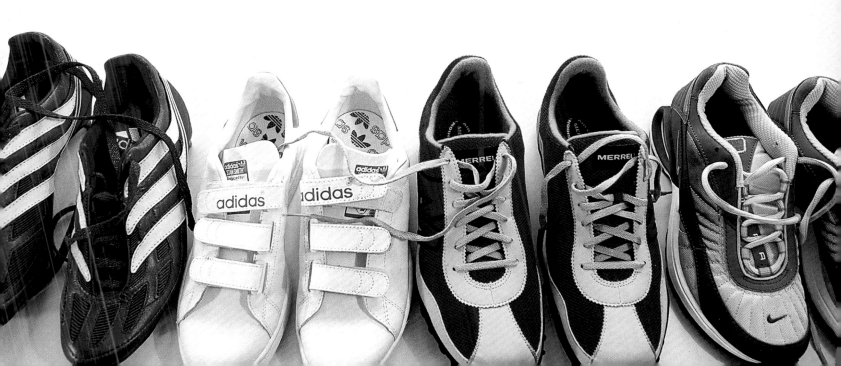

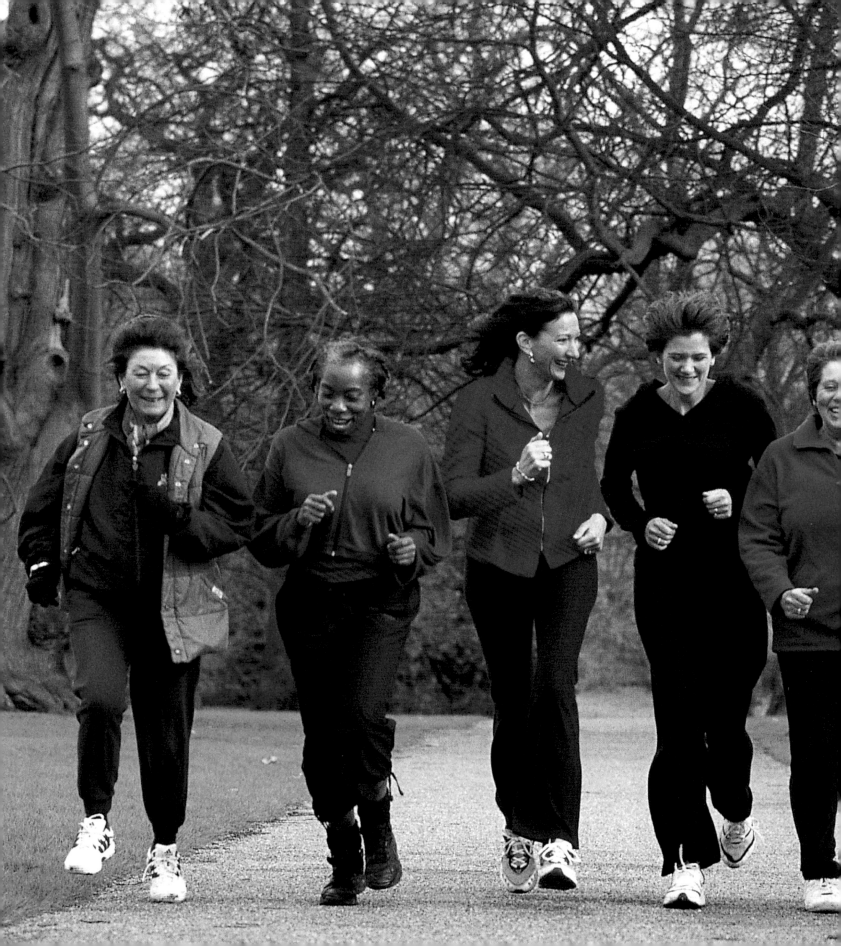

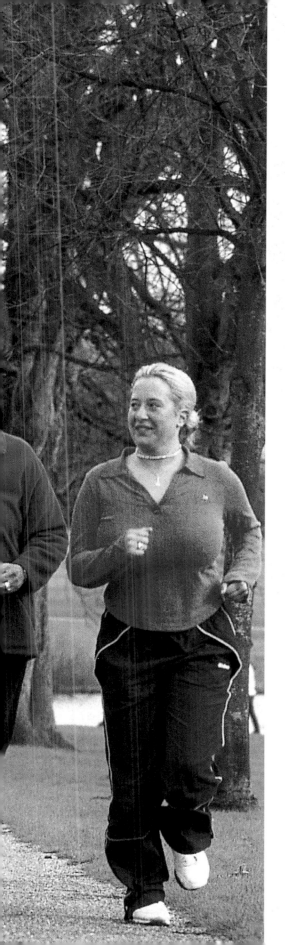

the exercisebible

THE **DEFINITIVE GUIDE** TO **TOTAL BODY HEALTH** AND **WELLBEING**

JOANNA HALL

KYLE CATHIE LIMITED

First published in Great Britain in 2002 by
Kyle Cathie Limited, 122 Arlington Road, London NW1 7HP
email: general.enquiries@kyle-cathie.com; website: www.kylecathie.com

ISBN 1 85626 420 3

Photography © 2002 Francesca Yorke
except: pages 13–17, 24–6, 28–9, 38, 41–2, 208, 214–5, 219, 222, 230, 237–9 supplied by Getty Images; 105 supplied by Mark Raudva

Editor Sheila Davies • Copy Editor Catherine Blake • Editorial Assistant Sarah Epton
Designer Heidi Baker

Joanna Hall is hereby identified as the author of this work in accordance with Section 77 of the Copyright, Designs and Patents Act 1988.

A CIP catalogue record for this title is available from the British Library.

Colour separations by Scanhouse, Malaysia
Printed and bound by Mondadori, Spain

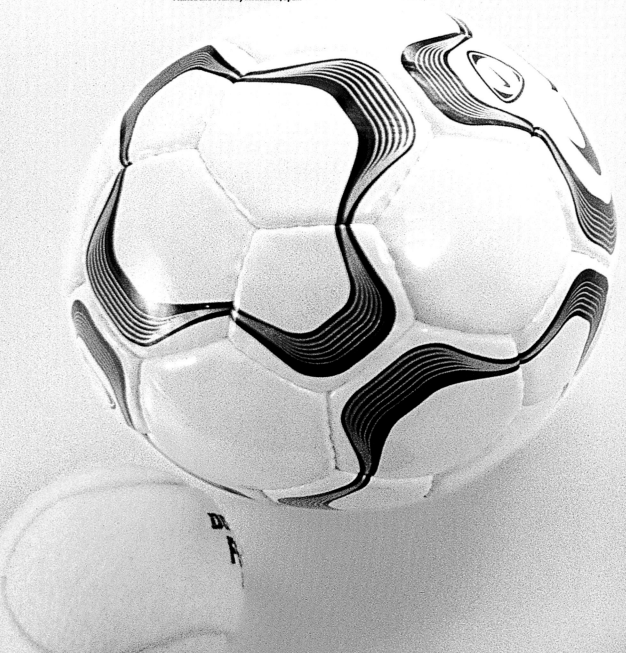

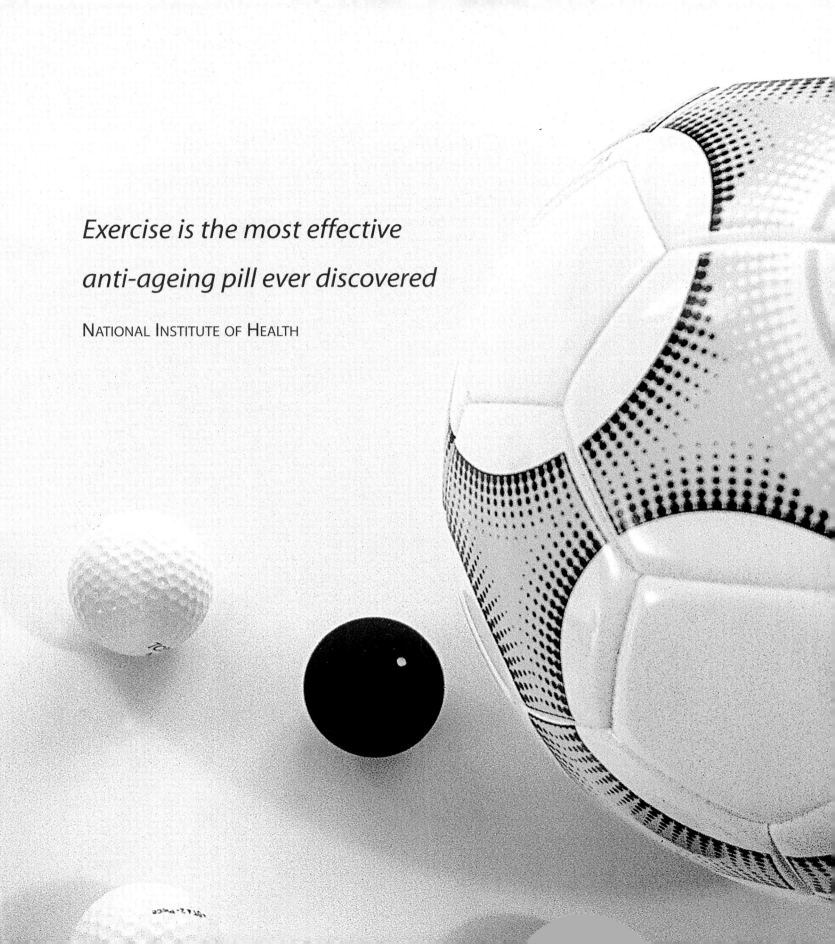

Exercise is the most effective anti-ageing pill ever discovered

N<small>ATIONAL</small> I<small>NSTITUTE OF</small> H<small>EALTH</small>

contents

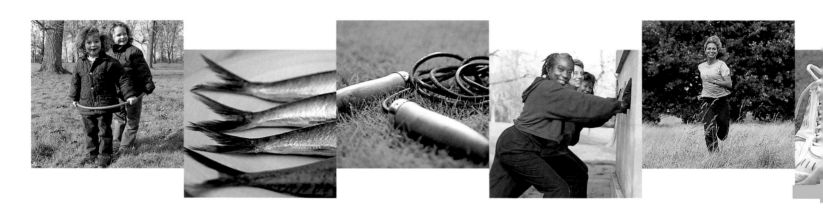

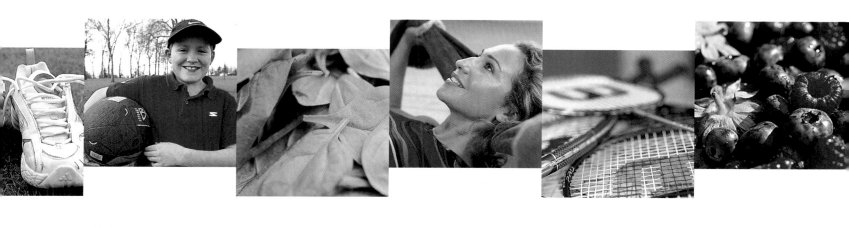

introduction

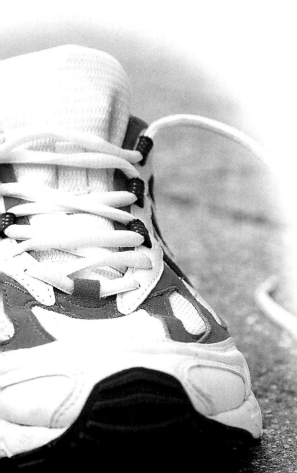

> 'Everyone should take their dog for a walk every day – even if they don't have one'
>
> Prof. Pers Astrand

I want to challenge the way you think about exercise.

Let's stop thinking of exercise as another thing on the 'TO DO' list and instead I'd love you to re-think how you can move your body.

So often we know we should take more exercise and eat more healthily but the perception of how much we have to do to improve our health and fitness becomes a pressure and not a pleasure.

This is why I have written *the exercise bible*. It aims to give you lots of ideas about improving your fitness, your health, changing your body shape, enjoying more energy and most of all feeling better about yourself. But instead of showing you how much you have to do to achieve all of these benefits, you'll find more of an emphasis on how little can you get away with and still get on with your life.

We live in challenging times. Times when we strive to fulfill our roles as individuals, parents, lovers, friends and carers. And times when we juggle our list of priorities with more pressing issues which takes away our time to invest in our own physical health.

Unless we take care of our body's health, the fragile life we lead can come to a grinding halt. If we want to keep the various parts of our life moving, we need to ensure that we look after the main cog – our bodies.

We all know we should invest time in exercise and that we need to eat more healthily but somehow something keeps getting the way – living our lives. Everyone is constrained by time but we need to change the perception that being physically fit and having a healthy body involves countless hours at the local gym or pounding the streets. Exercise is no longer just about getting hot and sweaty. The growth of the mind body fitness activities such as yoga and t'ai chi have enhanced our mental and spiritual wellbeing too.

The exercise bible aims to give you a one-stop guide to improve not just your health, fitness and body appearance but also your total wellbeing. It aims to provide you with the tools, information and motivation you need to understand and improve your body at any age, without putting your life on hold. Most of all it's about helping you to be the best that you can be whilst living the life you wish to live.

We now know there is a difference between being active to improve our health and being active to get fit. But this has created confusion about what we think we have to do and what we actually need to do to improve our body; so much so that when we decide to take action it is often difficult to know how and where to get started. The exercise bible aims to take away that confusion – bringing together exercise plans and physical activity programmes packed with lots of practical advice to help you achieve your best body whatever your available time, budget or needs. So whether you want to impact on your body's wellbeing on a daily basis, all year round or through your evolving life and lifestyle this book will provide you with a wealth of techniques, tips and practical information.

The exercise bible is not just about me preaching about this fantastic exercise or that technique. Yes, you will find great gym programmes and exercises but more than anything I want you to get a little excited about what physical activity can do for you. I want to challenge how you think about exercise. Small steps can help you feel better about yourself and positively affect your health, wellbeing and body. So I'd love you to share a little of my passion to see, feel and enjoy the difference. Most of all I'd just like you to

Be active

Joanna

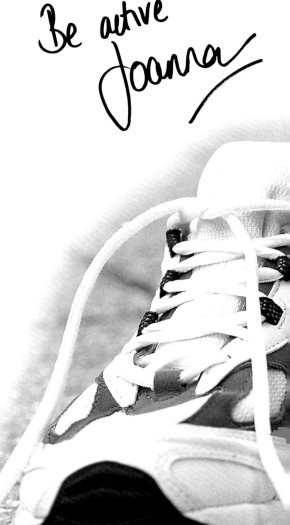

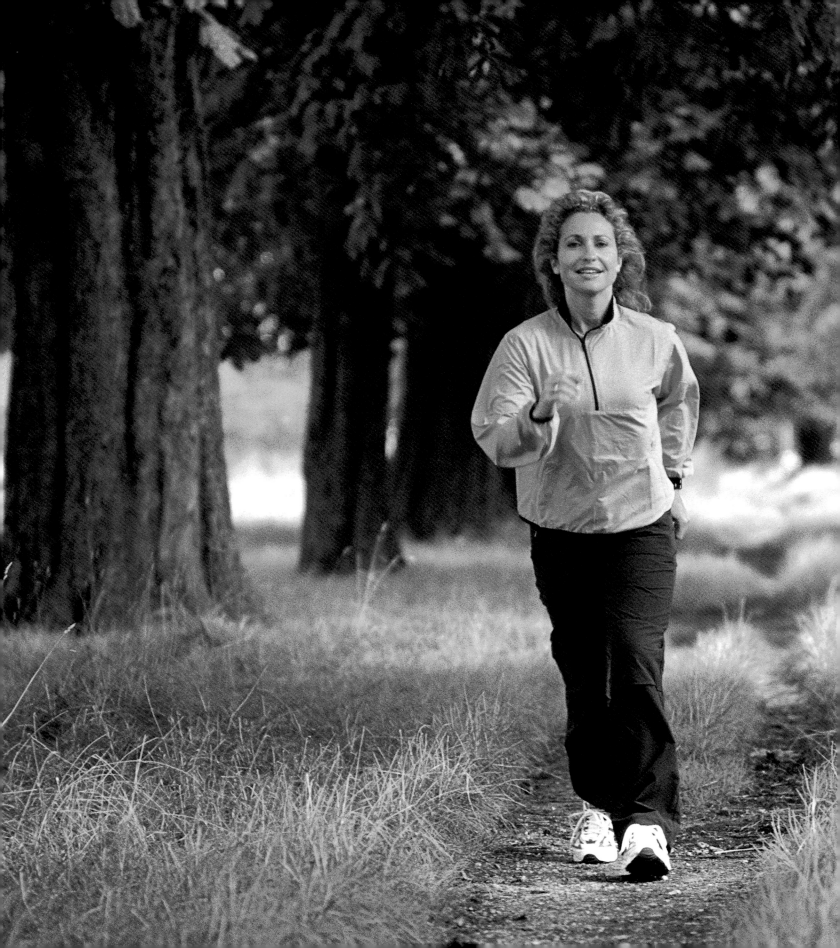

why exercise?

Exercise means different things to different people. It may mean sweat and tears on the rugby pitch, hordes of sweaty bodies pounding flesh in the gym, the lone runner crossing barren terrain, or just plain and simple walking. However, we all seem to be in agreement about one thing: we need to take exercise to become fitter and healthier. Exercise makes us feel good, improves our health, reduces our stress and slows down the ageing process – and to enjoy the benefits it does not have to be as arduous as you may think.

So you want to get fit. But what do you actually mean by this? Do you have aspirations to complete the London Marathon, Hike up Kilimanjaro, or does being fit to you mean being able to run for a bus without getting out of breath or not feeling exhausted after playing with your children for an afternoon? Fitness means different things to different people but underlying everything is the desire to have a healthy body. You don't have to be able to run a half marathon to enjoy good health – total wellbeing is a combination of mind and body. If you are motivated to lose a little weight, reduce your blood pressure, or your risk of heart disease, stroke and some cancers then the best thing you can do is start being active.

Ditch the 'no pain, no gain' mantra

Exercising moderately can be just as good, and sometimes better!

Most people dislike the concept of exercise as they believe they have to do it vigorously and to the point of pain to see or experience an improvement. If this is you, here are three reasons why you can should kick the 'no pain, no gain' mantra into touch and get moving.

1. **Lower-intensity exercise reduces the risk of injury to the skeletal system.**
2. **People with heart disease are more prone to heart attacks with vigorous exercise.**
3. **More moderate exercise improves health by reducing blood fats and blood pressure.**

The health benefits of an active lifestyle

Even more encouraging is the emerging evidence that moderate exercise can provide significant health benefits for people who are currently inactive. New health-related guidelines highlight the importance of 30 minutes or more of physical activity at least 3 times per week. This is the equivalent to a brisk walk of a total of 7–9km/5–6 miles for most healthy adults. Whatever your age or circumstances, exercise is a physical investment well worth making.

 Exercise protects post-menopausal women against diabetes.
Studies found that women between the ages of 55 and 69 who exercised regularly were 31% less likely to develop diabetes than those who did not. And if you exercise moderately or vigorously more than 4 times a week, the news is even better – your risk of diabetes is half that of women who rarely or never exercise at these levels.

To achieve these benefits, you don't even need to do your exercise all in one go. If you are juggling many things in your life, this great news for you, as you can improve your health without having to spend hours in the gym or pounding the pavement.

 Small bouts of exercise reduce cholesterol levels.
In tests, people who exercised for 3 10-minute sessions a day showed greater improvements in blood cholesterol levels than those who exercised for half an hour in a single session. See page 156 for the Cholesterol-Lowering Plan.

Regular aerobic exercise reduces blood pressure.
Studies show that regular aerobic exercise reduces systolic and diastolic blood pressure by about 10mm Hg. A word of caution, though: if your resting blood pressure exceeds 200/105, you should not take part in an aerobic exercise session. If you do not know your blood pressure, check with your GP. See page 156 for tips to reduce blood pressure.

Exercise alleviates depression.
Research suggests that exercise generally improves mood, and regular, moderate exercise has been found to be as effective as medication and psychotherapy in combating depression. You don't have to break a sweat to get mood-enhancing benefits from exercise – even a 20-minute walk in woodland and open spaces can reduce stress and change brainwave

frequency to the more stress-reducing alpha waves.

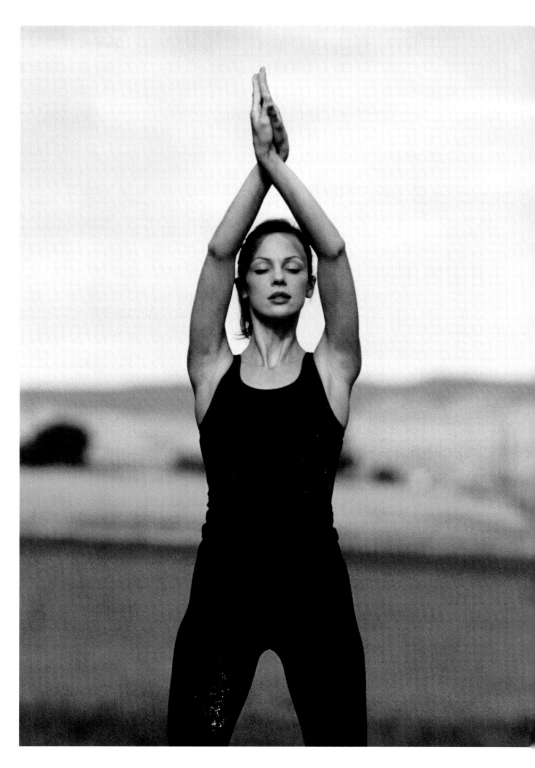

FACT **Physical activity reduces obesity.**
Studies have shown that regular exercise is the key to maintaining healthy body fat levels. Achieving energy expenditure through accumulating physical activity – has been shown to be more achievable for overweight individuals than specific structured exercise sessions. The National Registrar of Obesity has shown successful body fat loss has been maintained in clinically obese individuals when they participate in regular physical activity that burns 4,000 calories a week. This is equivalent to walking 65km/40 miles a week. That is a lot of accumulated activity, but don't panic! See pages 43 and 166 for ways to build physical activity into a busy life.

FACT **Exercise improves glucose intolerance.**
Regular exercise improves the body's insulin sensitivity. Insulin helps control our blood glucose levels, but as we get older, our cells become more resilient to blood glucose, so it is harder for us to keep our blood glucose levels stable. This increases our risk of late-onset diabetes (Type 2). Regular exercise and physical activity can improve blood glucose regulation and reduce the need for diabetic medication.

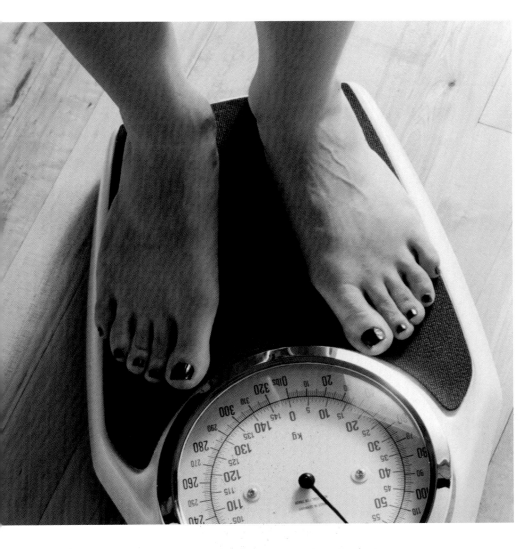

causing lower back pain (See the Better Posture Workout on page 102).

Childhood obesity typically develops into adult obesity, and also causes metabolic changes that make the condition difficult to treat in adulthood (see page 139–144 for getting and keeping your children active). Exercise – in conjunction with improving eating habits – is necessary to decrease obesity levels and encourage individuals to achieve healthy body fat ranges. Obesity management involves incorporating daily physical activity as well as the introduction of regular, structured exercise sessions. Throughout *The exercise bible* you'll find lots of ways to help get exercise to fit in with your life (rather than the other way around), so come on, give it a go! (See page 43 for tips on accumulating physical activity, and page 156 for weight loss suggestions.)

Body works

Our bodies are amazing. We were designed to move and be active but often we think we are more physically active than we actually are. Moving our bodies effectively for our health and wellbeing involves what we eat as well as what we do.

Obesity

Obesity is an epidemic that threatens global wellbeing. This may sound dramatic, but in reality 1.1 billion people are now affected, rivalling the number of people in the world who are undernourished and underweight. Health damage from obesity takes many forms: heavier body weight increases resistance to the heart's pumping of blood, increasing blood pressure. It raises the incidence of heart disease, strokes, breast cancer, colon cancer and arthritis. These diseases don't just affect you the patient, but also impact your friends and family members.

Individuals who are obese are 4 times as likely to have diabetes as those who are not. Heavier body weight also increases the stress on the joints, often

Muscle fuel

Although regular physical exercise can

improve body fitness, the quality of your training and the results you achieve will partly depend on the type of food you supply to your body's engine. Quite simply, food is fuel. But the *type* of food you are eating can directly impact on the quality and enjoyment of your exercise. We will cover this in greater depth in the Foods and Fluids Chapter (page 206).

Different fuels, different intensities

The fuels required for our muscles to contract depends on the intensity of exercise you are doing. Muscle glycogen is the fuel used for high-intensity exercise. The supply of glycogen, the storage form of glucose, however, is limited in the muscle, and when it is used up, muscle performance is significantly reduced. This means that long duration high-intensity exercise such as endurance bike-riding and long, hard running will be enhanced if you have more glycogen stored in the working muscles.

Fat is used as a source of fuel for lower-intensity exercise. You will be using more fat than muscle glycogen, for example, when you are sitting reading this book. As you start to move more and increase the intensity of your exercise, you will use more glycogen. But while you may be using a greater proportion of fat to achieve your movement at lower exercise intensities,

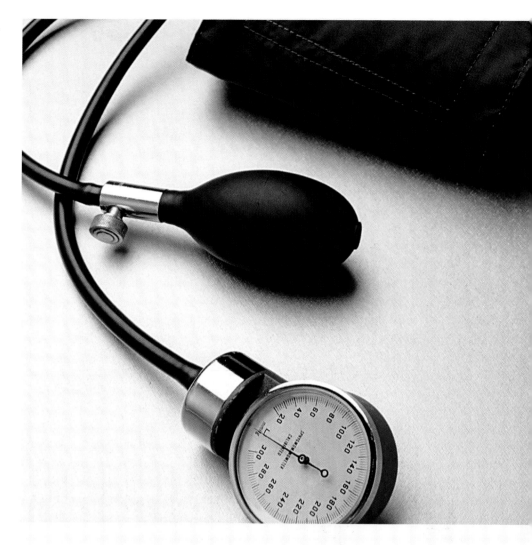

Ever got confused when your doctor takes your blood pressure and gives you two readings? Well, here is what it means: systolic blood pressure is the first number your doctor gives you, and is the force of the blood pressing against the walls of the arteries when the heart contracts; diastolic pressure is the second figure, and is the force of the blood pressing against the artery walls each time the heart relaxes. This pressure is measured in mm Hg. It is more important to monitor your diastolic pressure, because if this is high when your heart is relaxing, additional problems may arise when it starts to beat faster and is put under greater pressure to pump more blood around your body as you exercise.

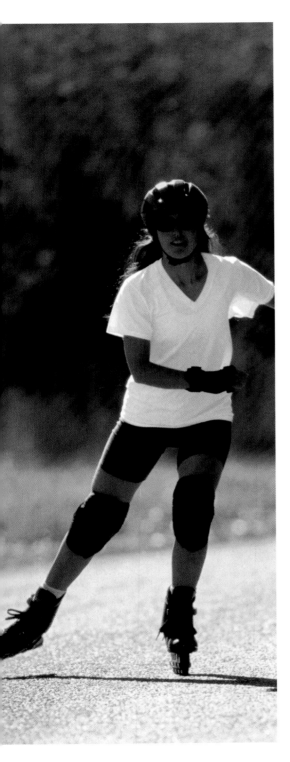

don't be fooled– the total amount of fat you are burning is small. If you are concerned about weight loss, it is important that you burn more calories than you consume, so you should achieve as large a calorie burn as possible. If you are short of time, the higher the intensity of your exercise, the greater the number of calories you will burn (see pages 47–8 for creative ways to expend calories in the minimum amount of time).

The Overload Principle

For improvements to take place, the body must be made to do more than it can comfortably manage. When this happens, the heart, lungs, circulatory system and cells are challenged, as they must overcome the demand placed on them. Physiological meachanisms in the body are forced to adapt and get stronger so that next time they can respond to the 'overload' more easily. This principle is crucial, for this is how our fitness improves; however, improvements in our health, such as reduced blood cholesterol levels and greater glucose tolerance, can be made without high-intensity activity. So we can eperience real improvements in health without having to push our bodies to excessive discomfort.

Specificity

The benefits we receive from our exercise will result from the particular demands we place on our body. This is known as specificity. Maybe you want to improve the tone and shape of your abdominals or pectorals, for example, or perhaps the cardiovascular stamina of your heart and lungs. To achieve a specific result, you will need to train that particular part of the body, stimulating it at a physiological level to get fitter, stronger and adapt to the training demand placed upon it. Without the training principles of overload and specificity fitness, improvements will not be felt and your exercise efforts will not be rewarded. (You can find specific training workouts for different parts of your body on pages 67–87, and training programmes for your cardiovascular fitness on pages 44–54.)

Variety

Just as your body needs to have specific demands placed on it, it must also have variety. Mentally if you are always doing the same thing you will get bored, switch off and lose your motivation. Your muscles can also get 'bored' if they are always doing exactly the same thing. They will stop getting fitter, and your fitness will feel it has hit a plateau. Having variety in your exercises (e.g. different ways of working your outer thighs or abdominals) and in the type of exercise (yoga, running, swimming, cycling, circuit training, etc.) is important, as it not only reduces your risk of injury, but also increases your fitness and creates a healthy, balanced body. This variety is often called 'cross-training'.

Use it or Lose it!

According to the Overload Principle, it is necessary to stress your body more than it is accustomed to, if a muscle is to achieve training adaptations. If a muscle is no longer stressed, it will 'detrain' and become weaker. Quite simply, you have to Use it or Lose it! This has an impact on both our health and fitness. Our bodies are living, active, incredible things which, like a car, are designed to move. If we don't move, things slow down, work less efficiently and eventually stop. To maintain our health we have to keep moving, and to maintain our fitness levels we need to use our bodies to the point of overload so that our physiological systems are continually challenged.

Rest and recovery

When we are physically active we need to allow our bodies rest to recover and benefit from the physiological changes that will be occurring inside. The analogy I use is with bread-making. You carefully prepare and combine all the ingredients, you knead the bread to strengthen the flour protein and yeast, and then leave the bread to rest and rise. It is exactly the same with the body – the kneading is similar to the exercise we do to strengthen our bodies, and leaving the

bread to rise is like getting rest and quality sleep. It is while the body is resting that it will be able to benefit from training. Rest, however, can also mean giving a break to different body systems or parts. Remember the old adage? A change is as good as a holiday! You could go for a long hike at the weekend, and *then* do your abdominals and stability programme (for balance and posture) on the Monday. Changing focus like this allows you to rest certain body parts while you can still work towards your long-term goal.

Daily activity

Of course there are things we can and should be doing every day. The benefits of walking have been known for a long time, but recent studies have quantified just how many steps we should be taking to develop our health, fitness and weight loss programmes. We can record the number of steps we take with a pedometer. (See pages 37–8 for more on pedometers and walking.) Our flexibility naturally decreases as we go through life and our posture become misaligned through daily stresses and long periods of sitting and standing. The postural and mobility workouts are daily programmes you can slot in to stop the onset of back pain and poor posture (see pages 99 and 102). As you go through *The exercise bible*, you will find may exercises that can easily be incorporated into your daily routine.

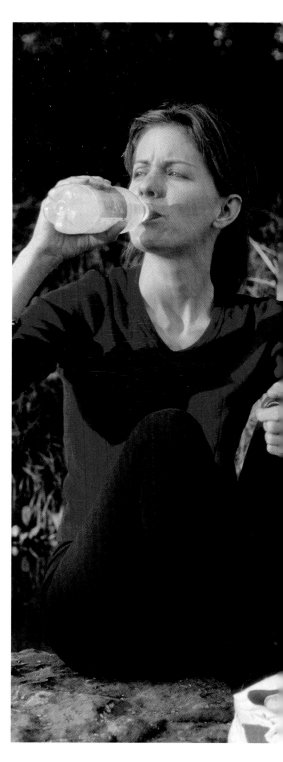

Warming up and cooling down

Let's get back to basics. We may be short of time, but if you are doing a serious exercise session you can't afford to skip a warm-up and cool-down.

Which movements are best?

Both for warming up and cooling down, any gentle movements that use the whole body are great – try walking, light jogging, gently paced cycling. When warming up, gradually increase your intensity – swing your arms faster if walking, and you will find that you can speed up your leg movements quite easily. By the end of the warm-up, you should feel you need to take off a layer of clothing. And remember, you can also do the Improve Your Mobility Workout (page 99) and the Better Posture Workout (page 102) to mobilize your joints, as well as some of the major leg stretches on pages 129–33.

The Warm-up

Before any exercise session it is important to warm up. A warm-up prepares us mentally as well as physically for the work we will be doing, and becomes particularly important when we perform more intense exercise sessions.

A proper warm-up should involve light aerobic work which puts your major joints such as your shoulders, hips, knees and spine through their range of motion. If you are tempted to skip your warm-up and delve straight in to the real workout – think twice! A warm-up is important because it:

1. **Increases body temperature.**
   Increasing your body temperature will reduce potential muscle injuries, as the muscle tendons and ligaments will be warmer and more pliable when contracting.
2. **Increases blood flow to the muscles.**
   The more blood reaching the muscles, the greater the supply of oxygen and glucose required for energy production.
3. **Increases blood flow to the heart.**
   The greater the supply of blood to the heart, the less potential difficulty there is for exercise-induced cardiac problems.
4. **Improves contractibility of muscles.**
   A warm muscle will be more elastic and supple, which helps it to be more mechanically efficient.
5. **Boosts nerve transmission.**
   Your nerve-muscle co-ordination will improve, which will mean better performance of certain motor movements.
6. **Prepares the cardiovascular system for the work to be done.**
   A steady warm-up will give your heart, lungs and blood vessels time to meet the demands of your workout. Without it you can quickly experience shortness of breath, discomfort and fatigue, as your body struggles to meet the physiological demands placed upon it.
7. **Encourages effective oxygen uptake.**
   Warmer temperatures in the muscle encourage the chemical combination of oxygen and blood (oxy-haemoglobin) to break down, freeing the oxygen for use by the muscle to produce vital energy.

The Cool-down

Just as it is important to warm up and prepare the body for exercise, it is equally important to cool down properly. A cool-down should involve gentle rhythmic movements and stretching.

It is important to cool down because it:

1. **Gradually decreases body temperature.**

   Cooling down prevents a sudden drop in temperature. Your body temperature will have increased, especially with cardiovascular activity. It's a good idea to Put on an extra layer of clothing to prevent body temperature dropping too quickly.

2. **Realigns working muscles.**

   Contracting muscles often shorten and need to be returned to their resting length to avoid a long-term reduction in flexibility and muscle tightness.

3. **Reduces the onset of post-exercise soreness.**

   Realigning the muscles helps to prevent post-exercise stiffness in muscles.

4. **Encourages blood flow to the heart.**

   During exercise blood is diverted to the working muscles. If you suddenly stop during intense cardiovascular exercise, this can make you feel light-headed as the blood is being diverted away from the heart and brain.

5. **Helps rid the body of waste products.**

   Rhythmic movements will encourage blood flow back to the heart. A greater flow of blood through the working muscles allows waste products to be removed from the body.

6. **Relaxes you.**

   Exercisers often report feeling more calm after exercise. A cool-down allows you to reassess your workout and have a few quiet moments to yourself before getting on with your day.

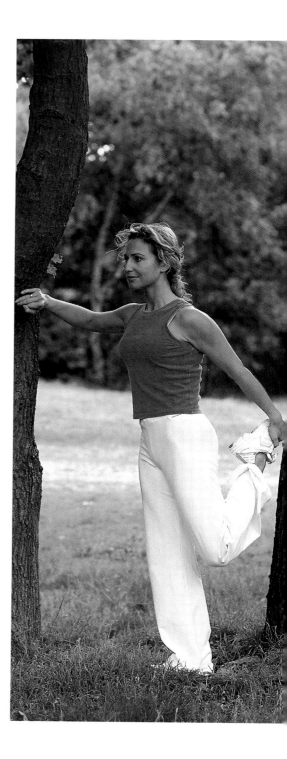

The 3 fitness components

We have seen how fitness and health can mean different things to different people. In the next three chapters we will see the importance of each of the three vital fitness components – whatever your motivation may be – and how they can be incorporated into a busy lifestyle.

Cardiovascular exercise

This involves the lungs, heart and blood circulatory system. It is also known as 'aerobic exercise' as it predominantly takes in and uses oxygen. At higher-intensity workouts the body is not able to meet its energy demands with oxygen alone. This type of activity is called 'anaerobic', and produces energy by breaking down other chemicals in the body. Aerobic exercise is beneficial to health and fitness, while significant improvements in fitness can be made when working at the anaerobic threshold (see A question of intensity, page 40).

Resistance exercise

Resistance exercise involves strength and muscular endurance work. Muscle tone and strength are important for good posture, improvements in body shape and enhanced feelings of self-esteem. Health benefits include reduced risk of osteoporosis, reduced loss of

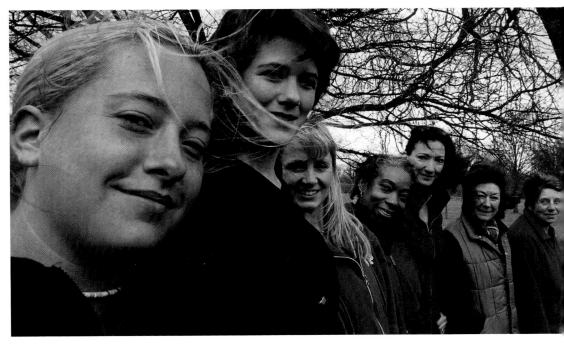

essential muscle tissue and increased bone density. The Best Body Bits workouts (see page 67) are particularly useful if you want to improve your body shape.

Flexibility

Flexibility is often overlooked, but it is an important component in our fitness and health programme. As we get older our flexibility, mobility and agility exercises can have just as much impact on our life as cardiovascular and resistance workouts. Whether you need to reduce your risk of back pain, improve your mobility when you get up in the morning or work on reducing your stress levels, you will find plenty of quick and easy-to-follow workouts on pages 99–135.

You and your body shape

Would you like to have a body like athletic Cindy Crawford, waif-like Kylie Minogue or curvaceous Kate Winslet? Well, if you want to look like Kylie but you look more like Sophie Dahl, the harsh reality is it ain't going to happen, because Mother Nature predetermined our body shape at an early age. In fact, Canadian geneticist Claude Bouchard believes our genes, together with the hormones we produce at puberty, determine our body shape by as much as 70%. So that leaves 30% of our bodies that can be refined, moulded and determined by what we eat and the exercise we do! According to a system devised by the US psychologist

William Sheldon in the 1940s, body types ('somatypes') generally fall into three broad categories, ectomorph, endomorph and mesomorph, each of which have distinct characteristics. There are very few 'pure' types, but although we may all have some element of each, most people will have a dominant type. Establishing our own body type is important to set realistic exercise goals.

So don't panic if you feel you are not a perfect size 10, identify your body type, and then follow the quick exercise tips to help you make the most of your shape and keep it in top working order. Remember, you can be fit and healty at any size and shape.

The body types

Ectomorphs – generally have a small frame with low body fat levels. They have an efficient metabolism and tend to burn calories off very quickly. They have a slim body shape, long limbs and thin face, and often find it hard to gain weight.

Endomorphs – generally have a more rounded body shape, storing body fat around the waist, hips and thighs. Individuals with this classic pear shape tend to have a slower metabolism, and can gain weight easily. Improving body shape can be challenging, even if they reduce calories and nutrient intake.

Mesomorphs – generally have a more athletic body shape with more muscle

Ectomorphs

Ectomorphs tend not to have a body fat problem. The main emphasis should be on improving muscular tone and increasing some muscle mass to help create shape, enhance bone density and reduce the risk of osteoporosis. Some studies have shown ectomorphs can suffer from depression and stress, so check out the stress-relieving yoga postures on page 168.

What is the best exercise for me?

Although excessive body fat levels are generally not a problem for ectomorphs, it is still important to be physically active to keep your body fat within optimum ranges. As a guideline, aim to take a minimum of 4,000 steps a day with a pedometer; studies have shown this to be the minimum required to maintain health (see page 38 to find out more). Mind-body exercise such as hatha yoga and meditation may be useful to help relieve stress and anxiety and to enhance flexibility.

Three Essential Ectomorph Resistance Exercises

Frontal Raise

What it does: Tones the front of the arm, specifically the long biceps muscle.
How many and what weight? The weight should be heavy enough to make the front part of your arm feel tired after 12 repetitions.
Want to know more? See page 89.

Abdominal Pillow Roll

What it does: Tones and shapes the waist area.
How many and what weight? Perform 20 of these. The longer you hold your legs and stabilize your abdominals, the harder the exercise will be. If you are new to exercise, start with the knees bent on the floor.
Want to know more? See page 192.

Straight Leg Lunge

What it does: Tones the buttocks and thighs.
How many? Build up to 12 repetitions for each leg. Use a chair for extra balance and perform them alternately at first to give your legs increased stamina. Build up to do all 12 on one leg and then repeat on the other.
Want to know more? See page 84.

mass and strong arms and legs. They are often naturally sporty and find their weight stays more constant, though they can be prone to over-developing their muscles.

How to identify your body type

A quick way to identify your body type is to encircle your wrist with your thumb and middle finger. If the middle finger overlaps your thumb, chances are you are an ectomorph. If the middle finger and thumb touch, you are probably a mesomorph. If the finger and thumb do not touch, you are most likely an endomorph.

Remember, all body types need a balanced programme for health involving a combination of cardiovascular, resistance and flexibility work. But each body type may require a different emphasis for each component.

Endomorphs

Endomorphs tend to lay down body fat easily, so they need to increase their cardiovascular activity to control their weight and reduce the risk of diabetes, high blood pressure and heart disease. See page 47, for cardiovascular workouts.

What is the best exercise for me?

As endomorphs are prone to laying down more body fat, they need to monitor their body composition. Cardiovascular exercise should form the basis of their exercise programme. If you are not a natural exerciser, it is a good idea to try a variety of activities to find the one you like, such as swimming, group sports or brisk walking (train to achieve a step count of 10,000 a day with a pedometer)? Remember not to be too quick to finish your workout, as you do need to stretch, too. To find out which muscles to stretch, see pages 129–135.

Three Essential Endomorph Resistance Exercises

Single Leg Press

What it does: Tones the front and back thigh, buttock and calf.
How many? Do 16–20 on each side.
Want to know more? See page 83.

Toe Touch

What it does: Tones and flattens the abdominal muscles.
How many? Build up to 12 with each leg. This is a subtle exercise, and if done effectively has great results when it comes to flattening the abdominals. If you have a back problem, stretch your legs out, keeping your feet on the floor, and then bring the leg back in again.
Want to know more? See page 79.

Buttock Raise

What it does: Lifts the bottom area.
How many? Perform 16–20 lifts and then 10 pulses. Repeat on both legs.
Want to know more? See page 187.

Mesomorphs

Studies have shown that mesomorphs are more prone to heart disease, so both aerobic exercise for fitness and resistance and flexibility exercises to streamline potentially overdeveloped muscles are a priority.

What is the best exercise for me?

Mesomorphs tend to be natural exercisers and are generally more active. To maintain fitness, 7,000 steps a day is a good pedometer-walking target. Flexibility and stability work is important to mesomorphs, as they are often susceptible to injuries as a consequence of trying such a wide variety of exercises. Ashtanga yoga with its more physical demands may well appeal to mesomorphs.

Three Essential Mesomorph Resistance Exercises

Scissors

What it does: Tones and lengthens the back of the arms.

How many? 20 each side. This is a subtle exercise, and when done effectively produces great results in streamlining the back of the arms.

Want to know more? See page 72.

Ball Offering

What it does: Pulls in and defines waist area.

How many? Build up to 16–20 reps on each side, making sure that you draw the opposite hip and rib together.

Want to know more? See page 81.

Standing Leg Circle

What it does: Firms the bottom and lengthens the leg.

How many and what weight? Perform 20 on each leg.

Want to know more? See page 76.

Top tips

1. To see an improvement in your body shape you need to use a sufficiently heavy weight, so that by the end of your prescribed repetitions your muscles are telling you they really don't want to do many more of that specific exercise. This feeling of overload is called 'near fatigue'. It is important to reach this point so that your muscles get toned. See page 62 for more details.

2. If you don't have hand weights, you can use water bottles filled with tap water. Of course, the bigger the bottle, the heavier the weight, so experiment with 500ml/18fl oz as well as 1 litre/1^3/$_4$ pint and 1.5 litre/2^1/$_2$ pint bottles to find the right weight for you. See page 66 for other exercise equipment ideas.

3. Never compromise your technique, as it is quality not quantity that gets you the results you want.

4. If you are new to exercise, always check with your GP before starting a fitness programme – especially if you have any medical conditions such as high blood pressure or joint problems.

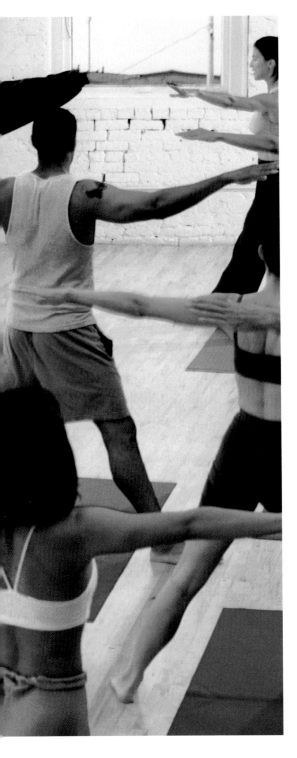

Motivation Checklist

How ready are you? You may know that you need to get a bit more movement into your life – but now motivated are you? Answer 'yes' or 'no' to the following questions:

	yes	no
Are you willing to set aside at least 10 minutes of your time each day to exercise?	☐	☐
Are you willing to tell others you are working towards a healthier you?	☐	☐
Are you ready to make exercise appointments with yourself in your diary and keep them sacred?	☐	☐
Are you excited about the idea of feeling fitter, healthier and more physically confident?	☐	☐
Do you realize that exercising may not always be something you want to do?	☐	☐
Are you prepared to accept that there will be temptations that will try to lure you away from your good intentions?	☐	☐
If you *do* give in to temptation, are you prepared not to throw in the towel and give up completely?	☐	☐

If you have answered 'yes' to 5 or 6 of the questions, you are ready to embark on a more active and healthy lifestyle. You appreciate it may not always be plain sailing, but heck, you know it makes sense – and while you may not always like exercising at the time, the benefits afterwards are just great!

If you answered 'yes' to only 4 or fewer, your resolve is not quite ready! But don't worry! In this book you will find lots of ways to slot exercise into your life without it being a chore, as well as tips on improving that motivation.

Your Body Checklist

How do you feel about your body and physical activity?
Answer 'yes' or 'no' to the following questions to find out.

	yes	no
Are you active at least 3–5 times a week?	☐	☐
Are you happy with the way your body looks, given what is healthy and realistic for you?	☐	☐
Are you happy with how your body performs?	☐	☐
Do you feel as strong as you would like to be?	☐	☐
Do you have as much energy as you would like to have?	☐	☐
Do you feel physically comfortable in your own body?	☐	☐
Do you appreciate your body?	☐	☐

If you have answered 'yes' to 5 or 6 of the questions, you are physically fit as well as confident with your body. Use this book to learn different ways of boosting your enjoyment with exercise and fitness, and discover new methods to stay in good shape.

If you answered 'yes' to 4 or fewer, *the exercise bible* will show you a variety of ways to raise your physical self-esteem, increase your fitness and improve your health.

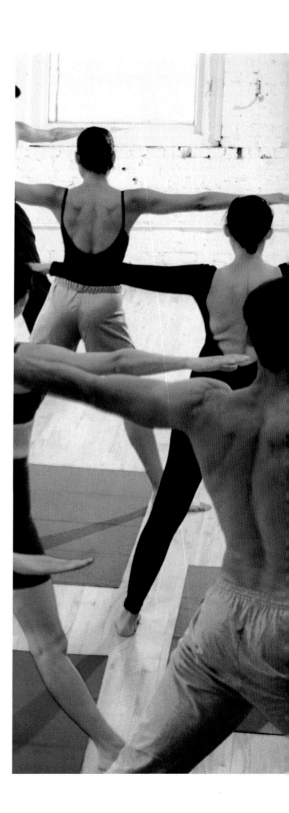

Your physical IQ

So you are ready to go – but what is your actual starting-point? Now is the time to give your body a bit of an MOT and find out where you are at the moment. Perform the following simple tests now, and repeat them in 6, 12, 18 and 24 weeks' time to see how you have progressed. Remember: fitness and health are not just about how many repetitions you can do in one session, or how far you can run, but also about how you feel. So make sure you record how you felt after completing each test.

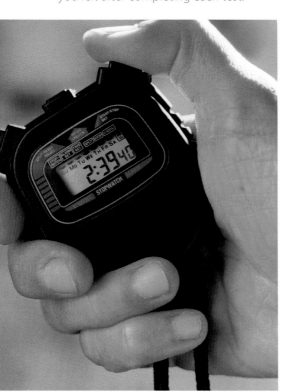

Strength tests

Upper Body Test

What you do: Kneel with hands just ahead of shoulders, arms straight and body forming one straight line from head to hips. Bend elbows to lower body until they are even with your shoulders, with your chest about 7.5cm/3in from the floor, then straighten your arms to push up to the starting point.
How many? As many bent-knee push-ups as you can (no time limit).

Lower Body Test

What you do: Stand in front of a chair, feet hip-distance apart. Cross your arms over your chest. Keeping body weight over your heels, lower torso until your bottom touches the chair seat. Take 4 seconds to lower and 2 seconds to stand.
How many? As many chair squats as you can (no time limit).

Abdominal Test

What you do: Lie on your back with knees bent and feet flat on the floor. Place hands at side of head. Curl head and shoulders off the floor, leading from the breastbone. Then lower the shoulders down.
How many? As many abdominal curls as you can in 1 minute.

Cardio test

The Cooper Institute's Aerobic Test

What you do: Time yourself as you run, jog or walk for 2.5km/1.5 miles on level ground. If you can't run the whole way, start off walking and gradually pick up the pace. Do you best but do not over-exert yourself. Remember to warm up before you start and cool down afterwards.

So how did you fare?

This chart provides a range of scores for the average woman.

	UPPER BODY STRENGTH	LOWER BODY STRENGTH	ABDOMINAL STRENGTH	CARDIO TIME
Excellent	33+	25+	48+	Below 12:50
Good	22–32	20–24	37– 47	12:51–14:23
Average	10–21	15–19	25–36	n/a
Fair	0–9	10–14	13–24	14:24–15:25
Poor	0	0–9	0–13	15:26 or above

Your Record

Date:					

STRENGTH

Upper body

Number of push-ups:					
How I felt afterwards:					

Lower body

Number of squats:					
How I felt afterwards:					

Abdominals

Number of crunches:					
How I felt afterwards:					

CARDIO

Time:					
Working Heart Rate (see page 26 on how to measure this):					
How I felt afterwards:					

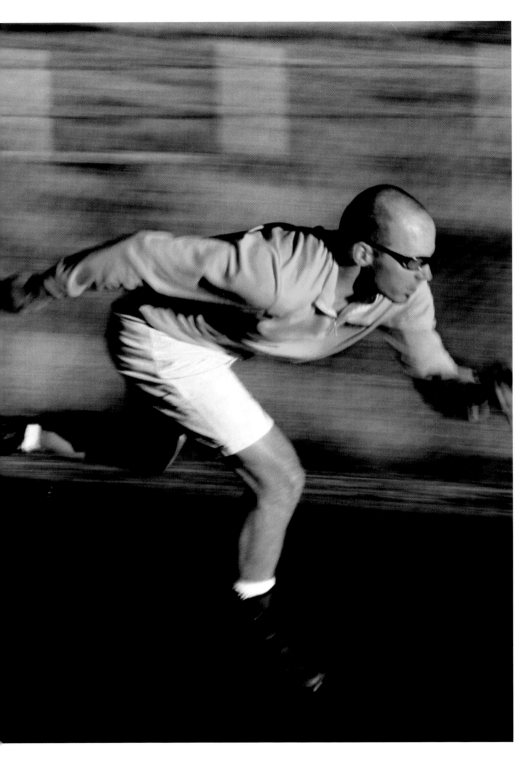

Body composition

Finally, whether we like it or not, we all need body fat and we all have body fat, 23 billion cells of it, in fact! The problem comes when we start to store too much fat in the body from over-eating and under-activity. Body fat gives us shape, warmth and insulation, but too much can increase susceptibility to heart disease, hypertension (high blood pressure), diabetes and some cancers. Too little and we may run the risk of decreased fertility and the onset of amenorrhoea, a condition in women when menstruation ceases. So before you start your health campaign, it is important to establish your body composition in the form of percentage body fat. You can measure your percentage body fat accurately with a body fat monitor, skin-fold collipes or with tape measurements. So what exactly are the healthy ranges? The figures shown below are broadly accepted as ideal:

AGE	18–39	40–59	60+
Males	8–20%	11–22%	13–25%
Females	21–33%	23–34%	24–36%

Source: European Congress of Obesity, 1999

As we get older and our metabolism changes, we inevitably lay down more body fat in our fat cells. Unfortunately, fat cells cannot disappear, but they do have the ability to get smaller as well as bigger.

Following the exercise and physical activity tips in *the exercise bible* will help you keep within your healthy body fat ranges.

to reduce your blood pressure, or maybe you want to learn to relax and sleep better. If you are concerned about the health and fitness of those around you, you'll find exercise workouts for the whole family, including the kids (and not only for their bodies but for their brains as well – see page 142–3!).

And what you want to achieve today may be different in 6 months' time, a year on from now, or maybe when you reach the next decade. *The exercise bible* will be your companion as you go through life, to help you be fit, be healthy, be your best shape and most of all BE ACTIVE!

What do you want to achieve?

Now is the time to give a little more thought to what you would personally like to achieve. You need to be quite specific about this. All the workouts and tips in *the exercise bible* will help you become fitter, healthier and feel better about yourself, but what is it that you really want to get out of this book? Just as you may set goals for yourself in your professional life, so you may wish to set yourself some realistic physical targets. Once you have decided what these are, *The exercise bible* will help you achieve them, building your physical confidence and changing how you feel about yourself. Maybe you have your summer holiday to work towards and want to feel confident in your swimsuit. Maybe there is a local charity run you would like to take part in. Perhaps your doctor has told you that you need to exercise

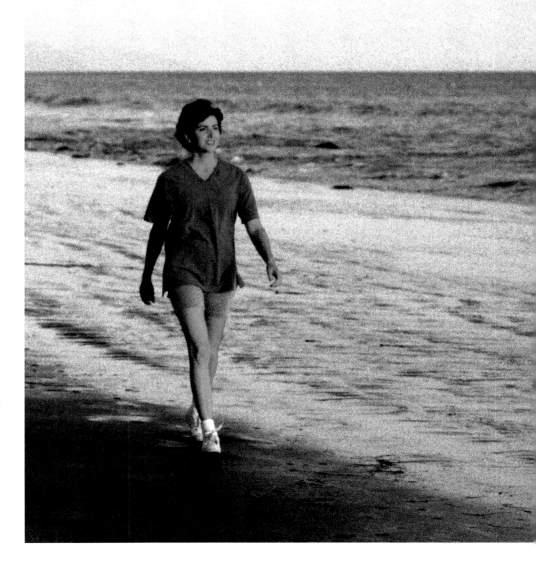

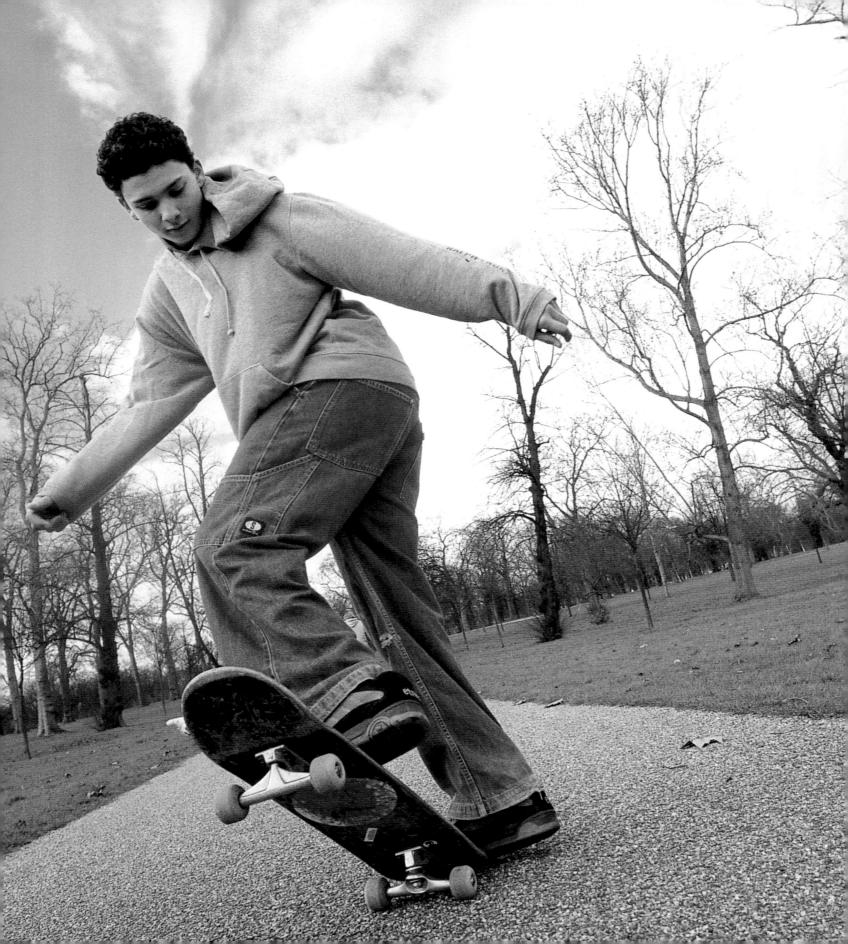

cardiovascular exercise

Cardiovascular exercise involves moving your body with the use of the large muscle groups. Often referred to as aerobic fitness, because it uses oxygen as a source of energy to create movement, it strengthens the heart, lungs and circulatory system. It provides significant health benefits and studies have shown that regular aerobic activity will add years to your life, and not just more years, but quality years – regular exercisers appear to have a greater sense of humour and optimism! So what are you waiting for? Get moving!

Cardiovascular exercise is any activity that moves your whole body. Aerobic or cardiovascular fitness may be measured by your body's ability to take in oxygen and use it to produce energy for work. You may still think of cardio exercise as aerobics classes and 'going for the burn' with Jane Fonda – but it has come a long way since then. Today there is a wealth of aerobic activities, sports and leisure pursuits that can provide your body with health and fitness benefits. Rhythmic, moderate exercise such as brisk walking, jogging, cycling, running, swimming, cross-country, skiing and rowing are all aerobic.

Why you should do it!

Cardiovascular exercise

- **Helps with healthy body composition.**
  Cardiovascular exercise helps your body burn calories. In fact, it burns more calories per unit of body weight than any other form of exercise. As a result, it helps to keep excess body fat down and to maintain an optimum healthy body fat percentage (see page 156 for exercise and weight management).
- **Elevates mood and relieves depression.**
  Exercise produces endorphins, the body's natural feel-good hormones. Studies have shown regular physical activity can be more effective at treating depression than medication.
- **Boosts your metabolism.**
  As we get older, we naturally lose muscle mass. Regular cardiovascular exercise can

help to maintain vital muscle mass as well as burning body fat, so that we maintain a healthy body composition.
- **Can alleviate PMS and period pain.**
  While there is only anecdoctal evidence, many women report decreased PMS and more regular periods.
- **Boosts energy.**
  As your cardiovascular fitness improves, your heart has to work less hard to do the same activities. You have a lot more energy and life becomes more enjoyable as everyday activities like climbing the stairs or running after your children becomes easier.
- **Reduces stress.**
  Cardiovascular exercise is one of the best ways to dissipate levels of the stress hormone cortisol in the body – so don't reach for the caffeine or bottle of wine without moving your body first!
- **Keeps you young.**
  What better reason to exercise? Regular cardiovascular exercise staves off some of the effects of ageing, such as weight gain and muscle loss, and studies have shown that regular exercisers have a better memory. Keeping young does not only benefit yourself, but also your whole family and your ability to look after them.
- **Reduces risk of heart disease.**
  Cardiovascular stamina strengthens the cardio-respiratory system of the heart and lungs, reducing blood pressure and improving your body's ability to transport blood fats. So taking regular cardiovascular exercise can be one of the most important personal investments you can make.

Types of cardiovascular exercise

Here are just a few examples of cardiovascular activity that you may or may not have considered.

Aerobic dance

Back in the '70s aerobics was the form of exercise that got everybody moving. Choreographed dance movements to music were popularized by aerobic icon Jane Fonda, and the leg warmer boom was born. But if you're bothered by visions of lycra and floppy socks and headbands, don't be – that was then, and this is now. A well-constructed aerobic dance class provides a good cardiovascular stimulus to the heart, lungs and circulatory system, and a variety of step patterns, movements and direction changes, which reduces the risk of repetitive foot strike injuries. Look for a class that combines both high impact (movements in which both feet are off the ground at the same time) and low impact (movements in which one foot is always in contact with the floor). This minimizes the amount of force down the legs without compromising the intensity of your workout.

Capoeira

Brazilian in origin, Capoeira combines elements of dance, martial arts and gymnastics to create a cardiovascular workout that improves cardio-respiratory stamina, agility and co-ordination. Devised hundreds of years ago by African slaves on Brazil's plantations, capoeira is a formidable martial art, subtly designed so the slave masters did not realize they were actually training to fight. You can try capoeira in many studios as well as on Copacabana beach in Rio de Janeiro!

Cycling

Cycling can be a great leisure pursuit and with the increase in traffic congestion many commuters now use it as their primary way of getting to work. Cycling has also become more popular in the gym with the introduction of spinning – a group exercise in which an instructor leads a class on stationary bicycles through a simulated cycling workout, all done to music. Cycling is a low-impact cardiovascular activity – but remember, a lot depends on the environment. There is a big difference between cycling 2km/1¼ miles on the level or slight incline and the same distance free-wheeling downhill! Cycling down-hill or enjoying a weekend ride may not be enough to improve your cardiovascular fitness.

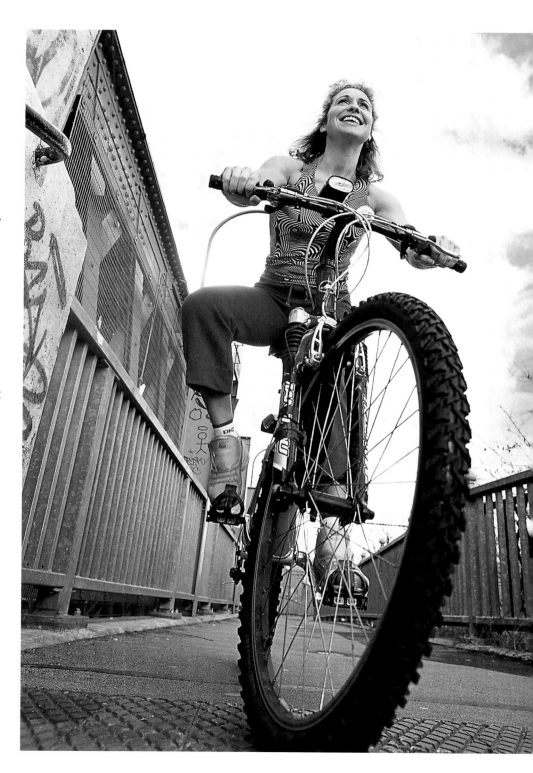

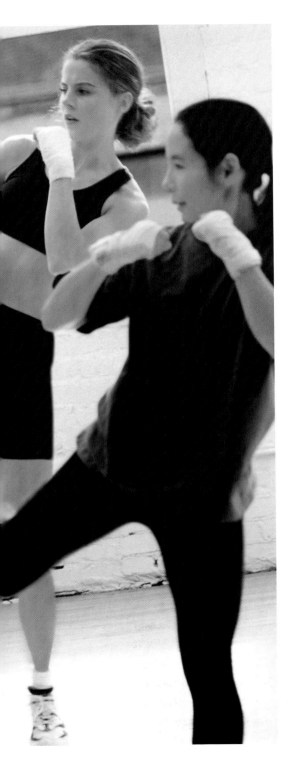

To ensure you enjoy each pedal push, here are some things to consider:

1. **To save you from a sore backside, wear padded cycling shorts. In addition, check that your sitting bones make contact with the rear of the bicycle seat. If you roll too far forward, the centre part of your saddle presses against the tender, soft tissue, causing pain and discomfort.**

2. **Introduce your bottom to the saddle slowly! When starting out, pedal a maximum of 30 minutes in total, to break yourself in gently.**

3. **Reduce lower back pain by maintaining a neutral spine position in the saddle . (See Rib-hip Connection on page 77.)**

4. **Neck pain worsens when you round your back and slump your shoulders. Retract your shoulder blades (keeping a good distance between your ears and shoulders) and stretch your neck at regular intervals during your ride. (Check out page 186 and 176 for shoulder openings and neck stretch exercises.)**

5. **Wrist and forearm pain can be caused by not maintaining a proper line between your forearm, wrist and hand. When they get tired, cyclists often 'break' at the wrist, placing additional strain on the wrist as it flexes, and causing the knuckles to lift and the hand to drop. Practise the wrist extension exercise to help strengthen the wrists (see page 203).**

6. **Foot cramping may occur if your laces are tied too tight, if your feet are too far inside the cages, or if you grip with your toes when you ride.**

Deep-water running

Deep-water running allows you to put in the miles and confront the same physiological challenges as training on land, but without the risk of impact-related injury. In fact, land runners have reported maximizing speed gains with deep-water training. All you need is an aqua-jogging buoyancy vest and a pool so deep that your feet cannot touch the bottom. Ideally the water should be a little cooler than body temperature. This will encourage you to work a little harder to keep warm. Burning 11.8 calories per minute, this cardio workout is challenging and not for the faint-hearted.

Top Tips
1. **When starting out, use a wall to help with your positioning.**
2. **The water-line should be level with your shoulder.**
3. **Your arm movements should be the same as when you run on land.**
4. **Flex and point your feet as you stride, as this will help with your stability in the water. It also helps to strengthen muscles in the front and back of the lower leg, improving muscular balance.**
5. **Hip flexion should reach about 60–80°.**

Kick boxing

Kick boxing, like tae kwando and karate, is a cardiovascular form of martial arts. It uses the lower limbs to lift, 'kick' and 'punch' opponents in a non-contact way. As the body is moving a lot of muscle mass, the cardiovascular benefits can be great. The self-defence aspects of kick boxing and other martial arts have made these classes increasingly popular, although they remain most popular with young people because of the range of motion and physical demands on the body.

Middle-Eastern workout

This workout combines elements of Turkish and Egyptian belly dancing that strengthen the hips, buttocks, thighs and abdominals. This form of exercise can have cardiovascular benefits and will also improve self-confidence, as it enhances self-esteem through sensual body movements.

Pole dancing

While pole dancing may be perceived as a form of activity to be enjoyed after hours, the muscular strength it demands, as well as the co-ordination and the continual movement of the body, can provide cardiovascular benefits and improvements in agility and balance. Pole dancing classes are becoming increasingly popular and devotees report a big increase in their posture and self-esteem.

Racket sports

Games such as squash, tennis and badminton are stop-and-start activities that place both aerobic and anaerobic energy demands on the body as the ball is played in and out. Although these sports have cardiovascular fitness benefits, the varying intensity of the games means that new exercisers may achieve more in terms of fitness by attending a regular aerobic session in the gym. In fact, as racket sports require bouts of high-intensity exercise – to reach for a drop shot or to run to the baseline, for example – it is better to build up your cardiovascular fitness before you start playing, with activities such as brisk walking, aerobics and jogging. As you get fitter, work on interval techniques to improve your cardiovascular stamina (see page 55 for details).

Running

Running may not appeal to everyone but it is one of the simplest fat-blasting aerobic workouts around. All you need is your body – and the courage to face the elements (in fact, running in the wind and rain can be quite exhilarating!). You don't need to be sporty, competitive or co-ordinated to learn how to run. If you can put one foot in front of the other, you can do it. The key to success is to start slowly – and I mean slowly. Alternate between walking and jogging (see the 'I can't run! How do I start?' workout, page 58) and in a matter of weeks you will feel a big improvement in your cardiovascular fitness. Running burns more calories than just about any other form of exercise; even at a slow pace it burns an average of 4.2 calories per hour for every 450g/1lb of bodyweight. (So, if you weigh 65.3kg/10st 4lb you will burn 605 calories per hour.) That is more than you will use cycling at 16km/10 miles per hour (2.7 calories per 450g/1lb), skipping (3.8), swimming a slow crawl (3.5) or weight training (1.9).

Running is a high-impact activity and the impact felt through your legs is consequently higher than walking, where one foot is always in contact with the ground. It may, therefore, not be suitable for everyone – if you are in any doubt, check with a physiotherapist, personal trainer or sports medic. According to some people there are only three types of runners – the runner who is about to get injured, the runner who is injured and the runner who's recovering from an injury! Yes, running can receive bad press because of the number of injuries associated with it, but often it is not the pursuit itself that creates the problems but the running technique, misalignment or wrong shoes (see page 236 for equipment guidelines and page 202 for injury prevention exercises). Here are some top tips to keep you injury-free:

1. **Try to run on a firm surface without camber, potholes or ruts. If you run on roads against the traffic, the slant of the camber causes the inside foot to roll in (supination) and the outside one to roll outwards (pronation). Both of these are potential causes of injury. The best surface is probably a dirt track. It is easy on the**

body and you don't have to watch continually for traffic. Get hold of a local Ordnance Survey map to find some interesting routes.

2. **If you are going for long runs, measure them in time rather than distance, as this will curb any urge you may have to push yourself the whole time to beat your personal best. Running should not be about competing with yourself each time you go out.**

3. **Change your shoes regularly. As shoes wear, the internal cushioning and stability decreases. Remember, a shoe may still look in good condition but its absorbency qualities may have significantly decreased. Aim to replace your shoes every 650–800km/400–500 miles.**

4. **Introduce speedwork to increase your cardiovascular fitness, but do not introduce it too quickly. If you do, you are inviting injuries. (See the sample workout, page 58.)**

5. **Work to the training principle of 'easy one day, hard the next'. You may feel great after a long, hard run, but remember your muscles will need rest to repair and replenish the muscle glycogen. Follow hard-run days with a recovery light-run day or rest day.**

What is a heart-rate monitor?

A good heart-rate monitor enables you to record how hard your heart is working and thereby helps you train at the right intensity. You wear a chest strap and watch, and your exercising heart rate is recorded using telemetry. As you get better at using the monitor, it will provide essential feedback on your hydration status and your levels of fatigue, allowing you to train more effectively and safely. Worth getting? YES.

Step aerobics

Step aerobics hit the fitness industry in a big way at the start of the 1990s. Involving choreographed steps to music up on to a block, step aerobics offered an effective cardiovascular workout while avoiding the potential problems associated with traditional high-impact aerobics. As step aerobics evolved, there was a trend to raise the step height, increase the music speed or introduce more complex choreography in order to provide greater challenges for regular class attendees. Unfortunately, as a consequence, step became the second highest injury-producing form of group exercise after high-impact aerobics. Nevertheless, with correct step height and speed it can be a very effective cardiovascular workout – particularly for the lower body: the fixed step height means that you can't cheat! Here are just five simple tips that can ensure your step workout is safe.

- **Check your instructor is getting you to step up at a music speed of 120–136 beats per minute. This means that you will be stepping up and down 20–24 times per minute. Any faster than that and you could compromise your stepping technique and possibly injure yourself.**

- **Watch knee alignment. As you step up, ensure that you extend through the knee and keep the mid-line of the patella (knee cap) in line with the second toe.**

- **Adding blocks to your step can increase the intensity of your workout by 12–15%, but check your knee angle does not exceed 90°.**

- **Change the step angle and approach to your step. This will give greater variety to your joint action and thereby reduce the risk of over-use injuries.**

- **As you step down stay close to the board to reduce over-extension of the Achilles tendon.**

Swimming

Swimming is an aerobic activity that uses the whole body, and therefore its benefits are felt throughout your entire system. It provides a great way to increase your cardiovascular stamina without the impact risks of land training. And if you are not a swimmer, aqua aerobics can be a good alternative (see the Water Workout on page 49). Moving through water in a position of least resistance gives buoyancy and support to injured body parts. It can also, therefore, be an effective medium if you are new to exercise or have joint (or potential joint) problems. Swimming is also a particularly effective and therapeutic form of activity if you suffer from osteoarthritis or rheumatoid arthritis.

Team sports

Team sports such as soccer, rugby, netball, hockey and volleyball are great ways to keep fit and healthy while enjoying the camaraderie and companionship of others. Like racket sports, team sports are stop-and-start activities, requiring both aerobic and anaerobic stamina. In addition, different types of cardiovascular fitness are needed, depending upon the position you play. Forwards should have more explosive-sprint anaerobic fitness while mid-fielders are more reliant on cardiovascular stamina, as they continually move to follow the play. It is important to build up cardiovascular fitness first, before concentrating on the specific requirements of your position.

Walking

Walking is probably the best exercise we can all do. It is the simplest, most accessible and least expensive form of exercise, *plus* it is extremely effective for the vast majority of people. Studies have shown that most people can achieve a training heart rate with brisk walking. It is an efficient low-impact cardiovascular stimulus, and an ideal first step towards a more active life. (To get you moving, check out the Walking Programme on page 44.)

The health benefits of walking have been known for a long time, but now research has quantified the number of steps we should be taking per day to

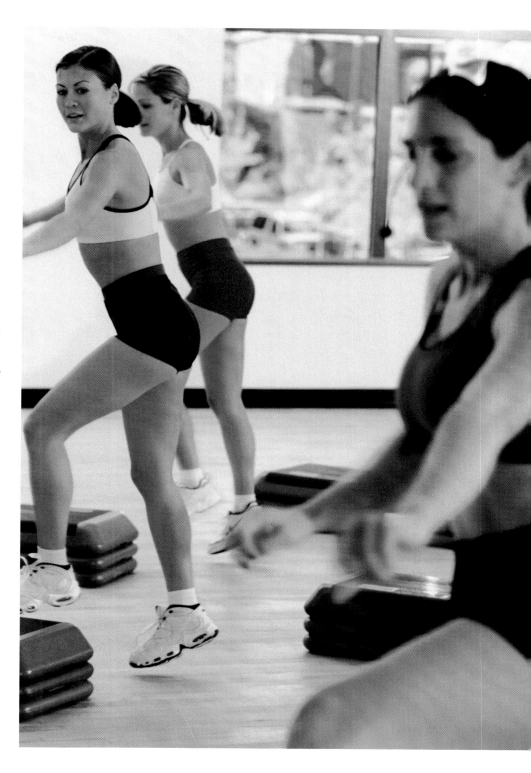

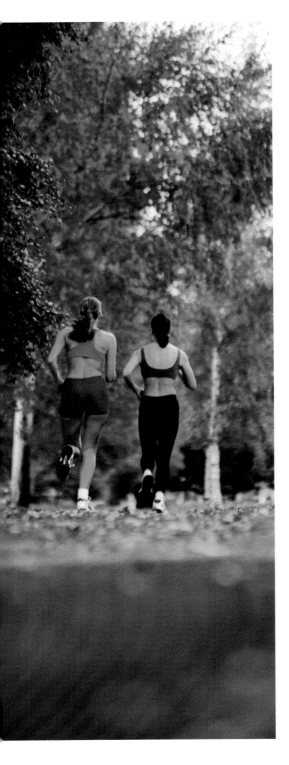

achieve specific activity goals. Studies show that we should all be walking a minimum of 4,000 steps a day to improve our health, 7,000 steps to increase our fitness levels and 10,000 steps a day to contribute to weight loss. This is really exciting as it means we can accumulate these steps throughout our day as we go about our usual activities. So what are you waiting for? Grab a pedometer and start walking.

What is a pedometer?

A pedometer is a simple device you attach to your belt. Calibrated to your stride length, weight, height and age, it records each step through a sensory device registering motion at the hip. Wear it all day to monitor your daily activity levels or to measure a specific walking workout. Worth getting? YES.

A word about safety

If you are exercising outside, particularly at night, there are a few things to remember:

1. **Wear reflective clothing. You must be seen by other road users. Many training shoes have reflective strips, and you can buy reflective strips to wear over your exercise clothing.**
2. **Walk or run facing oncoming traffic so you can see where you are going and be seen by oncoming cars.**
3. **Always wear a protective helmet when cycling and use bicycle lights at night.**
4. **If you are running on the pavement, have respect for your fellow pedestrians and let them know you are coming – and which side you will be overtaking on. It can be quite alarming if someone runs up fast behind you out of nowhere.**
5. **When road-running, lessen the risk of injury posed by the angle of the camber by varying your route and changing direction, so that both feet are exposed to the same degree of turn-out.**
6. **Exercise with a friend, particularly if you are a female, and let someone know your training route for extra safety.**

The importance of cross-training

Remember, with any activity it is essential to give your body variety. This can be particularly important with cardiovascular activity, where the same repetitive action can be continually channelled through a certain part of the body. Running is a classic example of this. Each time a jogger's foot strikes the ground, it sends a shock equivalent to 3 times their body weight through the feet and legs and into the spine. So try to vary your cardiovascular activity to compliment your existing routine. Here are some examples:

- **Running – try to add swimming. Why? You'll still get a cardiovascular workout, but without the impact.**
- **Squash – try to add cycling. Why? Cycling can build a strong cardiovascular base for the stop-start demands of squash.**
- **Kick boxing – try to add brisk walking. Why? The calming influence of walking will complement the more agressive side of kick boxing.**
- **Swimming – try to add step aerobics. Why? The weight-bearing demands of step aerobics (which are nil in water) will stimulate bone density.**

Body laid bare

And now for the science bit…

When we exercise, the body responds in various ways. While we exercise, it will meet the demands of that specific activity, and over a number of weeks it will adapt physiologically to our training. These changes enable us to get fitter, feel better and have more energy.

When you start an aerobic activity such as running, brisk walking or cycling, your heart rate (the number of times it beats per minute) and stroke volume (the amount of blood pumped out by your heart per beat) increase. Before you move, your muscles are at rest, requiring less oxygen. With motion, the muscles need a lot more oxygen. Blood carries oxygen around the body, so the heart has to pump harder to provide the exercising muscles with the oxygen they need. The amount of oxygenated blood that flows out of the heart is called cardiac output.

The oxygenated blood reaches the muscles via a fine network of blood capillaries. These allow the passage of oxygen and vital nutrients into the muscles, while waste gases such as carbon dioxide pass out – the blood deposits some of its oxygen, picks up carbon dioxide and then returns to the heart before going to the lungs. Within the muscles, tiny powerhouses called mitochondria use enzymes to convert the oxygen into energy in a form called adenosine tri phosphate (ATP). It is this that enables us to carry on functioning. Sometimes, if the demands of the working muscles are too great and the workout intensity is too high, there is not enough oxygen available to provide us with the energy we need. This condition is known as the anaerobic threshold, and when it happens the body works anaerobically to produce energy. This causes discomfort, and you can only do it for a short time. Anaerobic work creates undesirable by-products such as lactic acid. You will know when you are working anaerobically – you won't be able to hold a conversation, your lungs will ache and your legs will feel like lead.

The great thing about getting fitter is you will be increasingly capable of much more before you hit your anaerobic threshold. How does this happen?

Even within weeks of starting an effective training programme, what used to feel challenging will now feel much easier. The body has adapted to the demands placed upon it and a whole heap of changes has occurred. The cardiac output increases owing to an increase in stroke volume, which means that the heart is now able to pump out more blood with each contraction. A larger amount of oxygen can now be delivered more quickly to the muscles, facilitated by the development of more capillaries around the working muscles. And inside the muscles more mitochondria and enzymes are formed. All of which explains why, as you make exercise and regular physical activity part of your life, you feel fitter and your body is better equipped to carry on its every day activities. In terms of exercise, if a 9-minute mile/1.6km took your heart rate up to 160 beats per minute before you began regular training, that same 9-minute mile may now only raise your heart rate to 144 bpm. And when you are not exercising your resting heart rate falls, as the heart has to work less hard just to keep everything ticking over.

A few months of regular training are sufficient for you to notice the differences: you won't feel breathless when you run, or walk up a steep hill,

your muscles will feel firmer and you will begin to drop body fat. Then suddenly your training and the improvements will hit a plateau. Plateauing can happen for a number of reasons, but more often than not it is because you need to create an overload. If you don't push your training forward, you will eventually see a decline in your fitness (see page 16).

A question of intensity

It is important to monitor the intensity of your workout. There are many ways of measuring how hard your body is working, and some are more complicated and accurate than others. Whatever method you choose, it will make your training more effective as different levels of effort provide different training and health benefits. It can also make your training more enjoyable and safer. The intensity of your workout also determines how many calories you expend and the source of fuel you are using.

Serious exercisers often talk about 'training zones'. Training zones are levels of effort that create a training response in the body. Aerobic and anaerobic training zones relate to your degree of fitness and level of intensity. Aerobic training zones for an inactive person will be lower than for a fitter person. As

you get fitter, your training threshold increases along with your cardio output and your muscles' ability to extract and use oxygen. Aerobic training benefits generally occur up to work intensities of 80% maximum heart rate or 70% of your maximum oxygen uptake. Individuals working above these levels will be working anaerobically.

Heart rate increases linearly with increasing intensity, so an effective way to measure intensity is to monitor how your heart responds. However, there are several other factors that also have an impact on heart rate, such as caffeine consumption, stress and lack of sleep.

Below are a number of ways to monitor your intensity, ranging from basic to sophisticated and complicated. Select a method that you find user-friendly and that is most relevant to your situation. The table on page 41 summarizes these methods

Percentage of maximum heart rate

Exercise Intensity is most commonly expressed as a percentage of maximum heart rate. A woman's maximum heart rate is usually calculated at 220 minus her age. A man's maximum heart rate is higher, starting with 226 minus age. Depending on what intensity you wish to work at, you can determine your working heart rate. For example, a 20-year-old man will have a maximum heart rate of 206. His effective training zone would be 60–85% of his maximum heart rate. This translates as 122–166 beats per minute.

Percentage of oxygen uptake

A more accurate way to determine effective exercise intensity is by the amount of oxygen consumed as you exercise. This is known as 'oxygen uptake' or 'VO2 max'. Aerobic training thresholds are commonly up to 84% of your oxygen uptake. Establishing your oxygen uptake involves a laboratory test to analyze how your body responds.

Rates of perceived exertion

Establishing the correct intensity can also be done using the rate of perceived exertion (RPE).

When you exercise, your body experiences changes that are both physical and psychological (you will begin to feel challenged when you increase your workload). A combination of measuring both heart rate and RPE is considered by most people to be a useful way to monitor intensity. See the table below

Metabolic Equivalent (MET)

If you work out in a gym you may well be familiar with METS as a method of measuring your workout intensity. A MET is simply a multiple of your resting metabolic rate. One met is the equivalent to 1.2 calories per minute, so an activity that is 10 METS involves a calorie expenditure of 12 calories per minute.

Rate of perceived exertion

RATING	HOW DOES THE EXERCISE FEEL?
6	
7	Very, very light
8	
9	Very light
10	
11	Fairly light
12	
13	Somewhat hard
14	
15	Hard
16	
17	Very hard
18	
19	Very, very hard
20	

REF: Borg Scale 1973

Classification of exercise intensity (aerobic exercise)

This table shows a number of different ways you can measure your exercise intensity. If you are regular gym user it will be useful, as gym equipment often measure how hard you are working in different ways. Remember, you achieve significant health benefits when exercising moderately, and gain more specific fitness benefits when exercising at a higher intensity level.

CLASSIFICATION	% MAXIMUM HEART RATE	% MAXIMUM VO2	RPE	Young 20–29 YEARS	Old 60–75 YEARS
Very low	<30	<25	<10	<3.0	<2.0
Low	30–49	25–39	10–11	3.0–4.7	2.0–3.1
Moderate	50–69	40–59	12–13	4.8–7.1	3.2–4.7
High	70–89	60–84	14–15	7.2–10.1	4.8–6.7
Very high	> 90	> 85	>16	>10.2	>6.8
Maximum	100	100	20	12.0	8.0

Talk Test

If you find numbers and percentages a little daunting, you may find the talk/sweat test an easier option. Although less accurate than any of the above methods, it is less complicated, and a good way to appreciate exercise intensity if you are a new exerciser.

RATING	HOW IT FEELS	ACTIVITY EXAMPLES (depending on your fitness level)	SWEAT FACTOR	CHAT FACTOR
1	Very weak	Watching TV at home or film in the cinema, sitting in a meeting at work, sewing or reading a book.	No sweat.	Can chat to your heart's content.
2	Weak	Browsing in the shops, typing at your laptop, sitting eating dinner or chatting with friends, filling the dishwasher.	No sweat.	Can chat to your heart's content.
3	Moderate	Walking the dog, walking to work, playing a leisurely game of doubles tennis.	You feel a little warm in the clothes you are wearing. Starting to sweat.	Able to talk comfortably.
4	Quite strong	Climbing up escalators, carrying shopping up several flights of stairs, cycling for pleasure.	You need to take off an item of clothing. Starting to sweat on face and body.	Able to talk but not sing.
5	Strong: you are physically challenged	Mowing the lawn with a handmower, walking very briskly, pushing a pram up a slope, digging in the garden, light jogging.	You need to take off a layer of clothes to avoid sweating. Sweat felt on face and body – you will probably need to pop your clothes into the washing machine once you have finished your exercise session!	Able to hold a breathy conversation – but it feels a little uncomfortable.
6	Tough: you feel like you can only carry on for a limited time.	Fast jogging or running, carrying and lifting heavy objects such as furniture or weights in a gym.	Appropriate clothing worn to allow body to breathe. Definite sweating on face and body.	Able to hold a sporadic conversation with short pauses for breath.
7	Very tough: you have to force yourself to do this	Running fast to catch the last bus home, skipping with a rope, circuit training.	Body feeling very warm. Sweating. Light clothing worn to allow movement.	One-word answers.
8	Very, very tough: you are exercising at virtually your flat-out pace	Running in a competitive race.	Body feels very hot. Sweating felt during and immediately after activity.	Can just about give one-word answers, but have to catch your breath a lot in between.
9	Maximum effort: you can work no harder	Running for your life.	Whole body and head feels very hot.	Unable to speak.

Accumulating activity

By now you may be a regular exerciser, but don't neglect your basic physical activity levels outside your allocated structured exercise sessions. Think about it – you may be going to the gym or taking regular exercise for 60 minutes 3 times a week, but if you are inactive for most of the time during your day-to-day life, over the course of a week, that adds up to a lot of time of physical inactivity. Accumulating physical activity throughout the day has been shown to improve our health and this can have a big impact on our total daily energy burn. Here are the top ways to accumulate physical activity:

- Always take the stairs rather than the lift.
- Leave your mobile phone in the other room, so you have to move to answer it.
- Find something you do religiously each day and resolve to move your body for 10 minutes before you do it.
- Walk for 10 minutes before you open your purse to buy your lunch.
- Walk up escalators.
- Park the car at the farthest end of the car park.
- Get off your bus a couple of stops before your usual stop and walk.
- Always walk to the local newsagent, postbox, etc.
- Increase your walking pace by 10%.
- Walk to the next furthest bus stop rather than the one nearest your home.
- Use TV commercial breaks to get up and move your body.

The great thing about physical activity is that it can be achieved without you having to put on your gym kit! If you get into the habit now of being more physically active, you will find that it will be a great support strategy when life becomes a little too hectic to fit in every structured exercise session.

How do I know I am exercising at the right level?

Always make sure you can:

- **Hold a conversation with a friend.** This means that you should be able to have a breathy conversation with them – not talk continuously. If you can, this means you are putting too much energy into your conversation with your friend and not enough into your exercise!
- **Increase your washing load!** At the end of a structured exercise session you should need to put your exercise kit in the washing machine.
- **Strip off!** After you have warmed up you should feel warm enough to take off a layer of clothing. This will help your body breathe and prevent you overheating and feeling uncomfortable.
- **Do a little more** At the end of your exercise session you should feel like you have exerted yourself. However, you should also feel you could do just a little bit more if you really had to. You should not feel as if you have to finish on all fours, or feel queasy. If you do, you have worked too hard. Decrease the intensity at which you exercise next time. Exercising too hard will not be enjoyable, and it make you less inclined to continue with your new healthy exercise approach. It will also increase your risk of injury.

Getting started

Remember, you always need to do a proper warm-up and cool-down with all your workouts. You'll find information on this on page 18.

If you have any doubts about your suitability to exercise always check with your doctor first.

Walking Programme (5 weeks)

There are many ways to begin an exercise programme. Walking is probably one of the easiest ways for most people to get regular exercise because it does not require special equipment other than a good, comfortable pair of shoes.

This is a 5-week walking programme. If you find a particular week's pattern tiring, repeat it before going on to the next week. You do not have to complete the walking programme in 5 weeks – this is about you enjoying your exercise and increasing your physical activity levels, not just today but also in the longer term. Your aim is to complete a minimum of 3 walking sessions a week, and preferably 5.

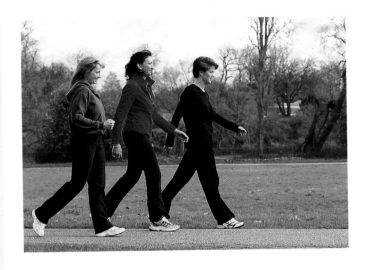

EACH SESSION	WARM-UP	TARGET ZONE EXERCISING; Chat factors 5–7	COOL-DOWN	TOTAL SESSION WORKOUT TIME	TOTAL WEEKLY WORKOUT TIME
Week 1	Walk slowly 5 mins	Walk briskly 5 mins	Walk slowly 5 mins	15 mins	75 mins
Week 2	Walk slowly 5 mins	Walk briskly 7 mins	Walk slowly 5 mins	17 mins	85 mins
Week 3	Walk slowly 5 mins	Walk briskly 9 mins	Walk slowly 5 mins	19 mins	95 mins
Week 4	Walk slowly 5 mins	Walk briskly 11 mins	Walk slowly 5 mins	21 mins	105 mins
Week 5	Walk slowly 5 mins	Walk briskly 13 mins	Walk slowly 5 mins	23 mins	115 mins

Beginner's Jogging Programme (10 weeks)

After you have completed your walking programme you may wish to progress to jogging. Remember, you do need to push yourself to maintain your fitness benefits. If you are a regular exerciser it may be more appropriate to start with week 3 of the jogging programme. To see the most benefit, try to do the programme 4 times a week

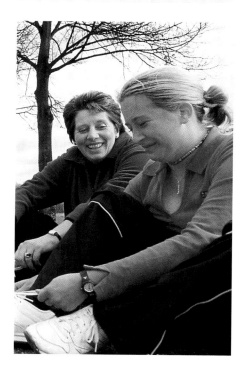

EACH SESSION	WARM-UP	TARGET ZONE EXERCISING; Chat factors 5 – 7	COOL-DOWN	TOTAL SESSION WORKOUT TIME	TOTAL WEEKLY WORKOUT TIME
Week 1	Stretch and warm up for 5 mins	Walk briskly 10 mins	Walk slowly 3 mins and stretch 2 mins	20 mins	80 mins
Week 2	Stretch and warm up 5 mins	Walk 5 mins, jog 1 min, walk 5 mins, jog 1 min	Walk slowly 3 mins and stretch 2 mins	22 mins	88 mins
Week 3	Stretch and warm up 5 mins	Walk 5 mins, jog 3 mins, walk 5 mins, jog 3 mins	Walk slowly 3 mins and stretch 2 mins	26 mins	104 mins
Week 4	Stretch and warm up 5 mins	Walk 4 mins, jog 4 mins, walk 4 mins, jog 4 mins	Walk slowly 3 mins and stretch 2 mins	26 mins	104 mins
Week 5	Stretch and warm up 5 mins	Walk 4 mins, jog 5 mins, walk 4 mins jog 5 mins	Walk slowly 3 mins and stretch 2 mins	28 mins	112 mins
Week 6	Stretch and warm up 5 mins	Walk 4 mins, jog 6 mins, walk 4 mins jog 6 mins	Walk slowly 3 mins and stretch 2 mins	30 mins	120 mins
Week 7	Stretch and warm up 5 mins	Walk 4 mins, jog 7 mins, walk 4 mins jog 7 mins	Walk slowly 3 mins and stretch 2 mins	32 mins	128 mins
Week 8	Stretch and warm up 5 mins	Walk 4 mins, jog 8 mins, walk 4 mins jog 8 mins	Walk slowly 3 mins and stretch 2 mins	34 mins	136 mins
Week 9	Stretch and warm up 5 mins	Walk 4 mins, jog 9 mins, walk 4 mins jog 9 mins	Walk slowly 3 mins and stretch 2 mins	36 mins	144 mins
Week 10	Stretch and warm up 5 mins	Walk 4 mins, jog 13 mins	Walk slowly 3 mins and stretch 2 mins	27 mins	108 mins

Once you have got the running bug and are able to run non-stop for 20 minutes you may want to work towards a longer distance. Now is a good time to train for a race or event, to give you a great motivational buzz. A 5km/3.1-mile race is ideal, and looking further down the line you may wish to enter a marathon. Both will require significant amounts of training.

You can use the planning below to help you put together a training programme. The number of weeks you need to allocate to training will depend on your fitness level, your availability to train and the length of the event. If you are already able to run for 20 minutes continuously and are new to running, 6–8 weeks training 3–4 times a week is a realistic time frame to enable you to achieve a respectable 5km race time.

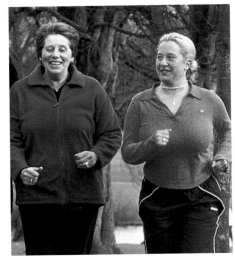

Typical week for a beginner's 5km/3.1-mile training programme:

Monday	20 mins
Tuesday	REST
Wednesday	3 x 5 mins fast
Thursday	REST
Friday	25 mins
Saturday	REST
Sunday	25 mins

For a 10km/6.2 mile event, you can keep to 4 sessions a week but increase your 'long' Sunday run until you're doing 60 minutes.

And if you watch running marathon events and have aspirations to complete a marathon yourself, here's a glimpse of what's involved. . . Once you have completed some longer distances and you are ready to tackle a marathon, you should allow at least 4 months to train for your first marathon. Often this will involve training through the winter months (see page 35–6 for information on equipment and saftey in order to train wisely and effectively).

A typical week of a marathon training (towards the end) will look like this:

Monday	40 mins' running at a steady pace
Tuesday	30 mins' speed work
Wednesday	45 mins' running at a steady pace
Thursday	60 mins (include 3 x 8 mins fast)
Friday	REST
Saturday	40 mins' hilly run
Sunday	3 hours' long run

With half marathons and shorter races, it is a good idea to complete the full event distance at least 3 weeks before the day of the race. This will boost your confidence and give you vital distance training experience. While it will not guarantee you a great performance, it will give you an idea of what to expect. With longer events such as marathons and ultra distance events, it is normal not to complete the full distance as the training schedule, correctly followed, will provide your body with all the training adaptations necessary to get you through the event. But remember – always listen to your body and ENJOY the physical achievements you have strived for.

15-minute Cardiovascular Workouts

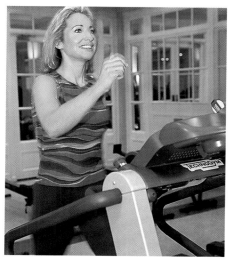

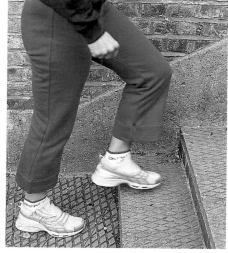

When you want to exercise but find yourself short of time, these 15-minute cardiovascular workouts can easily slot into your day, no matter where you are, or what the weather. Be creative with your time!

In the Gym:

Try this workout on the treadmill or any other piece of cardio equipment:

Minutes 1–4	Brisk walk
Minutes 4–7	Jog/run
Minutes 7–7½	As fast as you can
Minutes 7½–8½	Jog/run
Minutes 8½–9	As fast as you can
Minutes 9–10	Jog/run
Minutes 10–13	As fast as you can
Minutes 13–15	Walk

If you don't like the treadmill, you can apply this workout to any other piece of cardio equipment – rower, stairmaster, elliptical trainer, stationary bicycle.

At Home:

Minutes 1–3	Walk up and down your stairs or bottom stair. Roll shoulders x 8 right and left, side bends x 4 right and left.
Cardio circuit:	Do the following exercises for 1 minute each. Aim to work at an intensity level of 12–15 (see page 45). The fitter you are, the harder you will be able to push yourself. Step-ups on a step. Jumping jacks. Knee lifts. 30 seconds' active recovery – walk briskly on the spot or around the room to catch your breath. Repeat whole circuit from the top a total of 3 times.
Minutes 13–15	Cool down with a steady walk. Stretch quadriceps, hamstrings calf muscles and Achilles tendon. (See standing positions, page 129–132)

In the Pool:

Stick on your swim suit and aqua-jogging belt or vest and go deep-water jogging.

Minutes 1–3	Walk the shallow end of the pool 4 times. Roll your shoulders and stretch your arms above your head.
Minutes 3–12	Deep-water jogging.
Minutes 12–15	Repeat warm-up in reverse. Stretch calf muscles, quadriceps and hamstrings. (See page 129–132)

30-minute Calorie-blaster

The faster you walk, the more calories you will burn. The longer you walk the more calories you will burn. But it's hard to walk fast for long unless you are already in great shape. So here's a realistic compromise that will save you time and maximize the amount of calories you can burn. Intersperse fast walking bursts with more moderate walking. If you are a runner, then apply the same principles to your running on the treadmill.

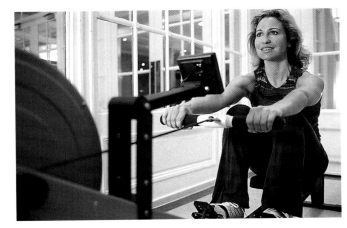

If you don't like the treadmill, you can apply this workout to other cardio equipment – rower, stairmaster, elliptical trainer, stationary bicycle. In fact, for a week of cross-training, aim to do the workout on four different pieces of equipment.

DURATION	In the Gym: TREADMILL SPEED	At Home: SPEED (if walking outside)
5 mins	2.8mph/4.5kmph up to 3.2mph/5.1kmph	Steady pace, so after 5 mins you feel you need to take off a layer of clothing. See intensity rating chart on page 46.
2 mins	3.8–4.2mph/6.1–6.8kmph	A brisk pace that you can sustain with relative comfort. You should be able to hold a breathy conversation with a friend.
2 mins	4.1–4.7mph/6.6–7.6kmph	A faster pace. You should feel by the end of the 2 mins you want to go back to your slower recovery pace as above.
2 mins	3.8–4.2mph/6.1–6.8kmph	A brisk pace that you can sustain with relative comfort. You should be able to hold a breathy conversation with a friend.
2 mins	4.1–4.7mph/6.6–7.6kmph	A faster pace. You should feel by the end of the 2 mins you want to go back to your slower recovery pace as above.
2 mins	3.8–4.2mph/6.1–6.8kmph	A brisk pace that you can sustain with relative comfort. You should be able to hold a breathy conversation with a friend.
2 mins	4.1–4.7mph/6.6–7.6kmph	A faster pace. You should feel by the end of the 2 mins you want to go back to your slower recovery pace as above.
2 mins	3.8–4.2mph/6.1–6.8kmph	A brisk pace that you can sustain with relative comfort. You should be able to hold a breathy conversation with a friend.
2 mins	4.1–4.7mph/6.6–7.6kmph	A faster pace. You should feel by the end of the 2 mins you want to go back to your slower recovery pace as above.
2 mins	3.8–4.2mph/6.1–6.8kmph	A brisk pace that you can sustain with relative comfort. You should be able to hold a breathy conversation with a friend.
2 mins	4.1–4.7mph/6.6–7.6kmph	A faster pace. You should feel by the end of the 2 mins you want to go back to your slower recovery pace as above.
5 mins	4.0mph/6.4kmph easing down to 2.5mph/4.0kmph	Gradually slow down so you can hold a comfortable conversation with a friend.

Water Workout

This is a really simple-to-follow water workout that can be done in a small pool. Water is 1,000 times more dense than air, and provides up to 12 times the resistance you can get from doing the same thing on land. Ideally the water should come up to your chest.

The aim is to do this workout, which will take less than 30 minutes, 3 times a week. Try to move more with each cardio set that you complete. Remember the more movement you create in the water, the harder your body works

So what are you waiting for? Grab that cozzie!

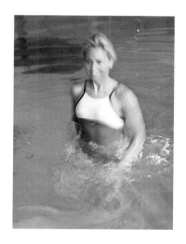

Water Warm-up (3–5 minutes)

Perform light, easy movements such as jogging. Press your heels to the bottom of the pool and practise sculling (making a figure-of-8 motion with your hands) for balance. Pace your warm-up according to the water temperature. When the water is colder, your movements need to be more vigorous. Gradually make them bigger and increase the speed. Move on to travelling movements to make your body work harder and to challenge your stability and balance.

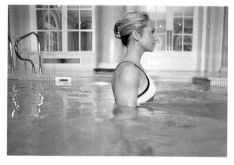 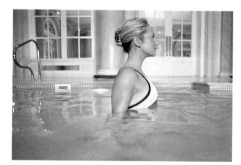

Muscular Toning Set I

What it does: Shoulders and upper back; great for posture.

How you do it: Begin with the arms in front, thumbs up and shoulders down. Pull your arms back, squeezing your shoulder blades together at the back, forming a back cleavage. Relax forward. In shallow water Jog backwards as you perform the exercise, to make your shoulders work harder.

How many: 12–20 repetitions

Cardio Work Set 1 (2–3 minutes)

The goal of each cardio work set is to make as much water movement as possible, to create more resistance.

What it does: Boosts stamina of heart and lungs

How you do it: Walk or run forward in a zigzag pattern across the pool. When you reach the end, run in a straight line backwards through the currents. Stabilize the body by keeping the chest high and maintain good running form by slicing with the hands and pumping the arms. Scull the hands in front if you need extra support.

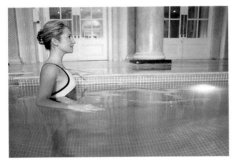 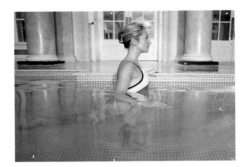

Muscular Toning Set 2

What it does: Tones buttocks and thighs.

How you do it: Begin with the leg at the surface, then strongly push the leg downward, so that it is fully extended. Relax and recover, with the leg bent. In shallow water you will be able to travel backwards as you push your leg back. Do not jump.

How many: 12–20 repetitions

Cardio Work Set 2: (2–3 minutes)

The goal of each cardio work set is to make as much water movement as possible, to create more resistance. Run forwards, sideways to the left, backwards, then sideways to the right, making a square. Then change direction. Repeat, altering the size of the square.

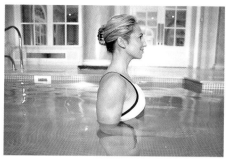

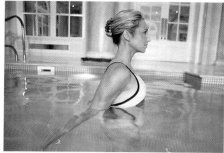

Muscular Toning Set 3

What it does: Tones triceps.

How you do it: Begin with the hand (palm up or down) near the surface. Push back, extending your elbow. On recovery, slice the hand back to the front and relax. In shallow water, travel backwards as you straighten the elbow. In deep water you can lift the body up as you press the elbow back.

How many: 12–20 repetitions

Cardio Work Set 3 (2–3 minutes)

The goal of each cardio work set is to make as much water movement as possible, to create more resistance. Run from side to side 3 times, then forwards and backwards 3 times, making the shape of a plus sign. Repeat the pattern, changing the speed, area and number of repetitions.

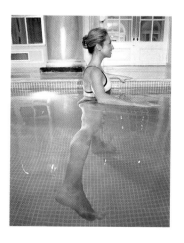

Muscular Toning Set 4

What it does: Tones inner and outer thighs.

How you do it: Begin in a standing position then power-push one leg to the side, toes pointing forwards. Let the body fall with the push. Relax as you bring your legs back together.

To work the inner thigh, begin standing with one leg extended to the side. Power-pull the leg to the centre. Aim towards working both legs simultaneously. Focus on squeezing the legs together. Relax as you allow the legs to part. In deeper water you may find holding on to the side of the pool helps your balance.

How many: 12–20 repetitions

Cardio Work Set 4 (2–3 minutes)

The goal of each cardio work set is to make as much water movement as possible, to create more resistance. Run a square. Reverse. Zigzag forwards then backwards. Turn and run a circle. Reverse. Repeat.

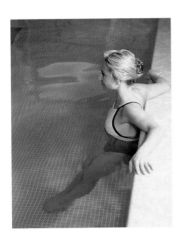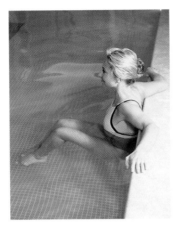

Muscular Toning Set 5

What it does: Tones the abdominal trunk muscles.

How you do it: Begin with your back against the side of the pool, holding on with your arms. Start with the legs together and extended straight down to the bottom, with your back in a neutral position against the side. Pull your legs in to your chest as you keep your back against the wall. The straighter your legs as you lift, the harder your abdominal muscles will work.

How many: 12–20 repetitions

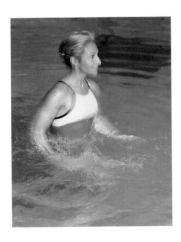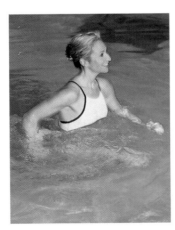

Water Warm-down (3–5 minutes)

Before you get out, perform some light movements that involve the whole body, such as walking and gentle jogging. Swing the arms forwards and backwards slightly out of the water. This will relax the muscles you have used and allow them to stay warm. Move towards the shallower end of the pool, so you will have the added benefit of gravity to help you recover.

Even Simpler Water Workout

If you feel the Water Workout is too complicated, here is something you may fancy instead. This is a really simple workout and can be easily done while on a summer holiday in a swimming pool with the children. Aim to it 3 times a week.

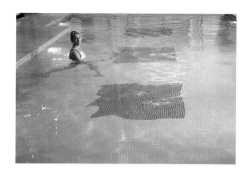
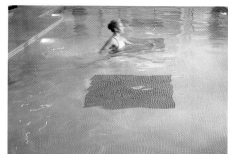
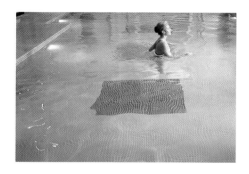
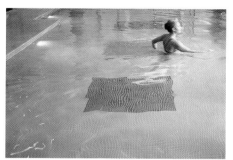

Perform your water warm-up as on page 49.

Walk across the shallow end of the pool 4 times. Take large strides and position yourself so the water is chest-height.

Hold on to the side of the pool and flutter-kick your legs for 30 seconds. .

Repeat the whole sequence 8 times for a simple yet effective cardio blast.

Top Tip: This is a great little cardio blast when you're on holiday in the sun with your family and you have to watch the children in the shallow end!

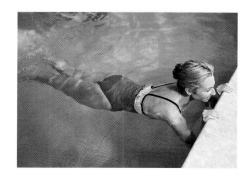

Swimming Programme (5 weeks)

Water acts as a giant cushion for the body. It is much kinder to vulnerable joints and tendons than hard surfaces such as concrete and Tarmac, and it can be especially useful as an exercise medium if you are overweight or suffer from joint problems.

The goal of this programme is to get you swimming continuously for 30 minutes, with 3 sessions a week.

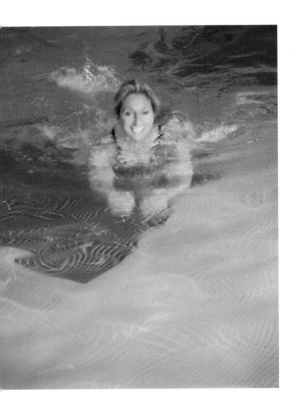

Warm-up

Complete a warm-up of 5 minutes with a variety of different strokes: try just breaststroke arms, flutter-kick legs and front- and back-crawl arms. This will increase the mobility of the joints and increase your body temperature. As with any warm-up, remember to start out slowly and gradually increase the size and speed of your movements.

Sessions 1 and 3

Week 1: Swim continuously at steady pace for 15 minutes. Change your stroke to ease any muscle discomfort you may experience through repetitive movement.

Week 2: Add 3 minutes to your swim time to complete 18 minutes of total swim time.

Week 3: Add 4 minutes to your swim time to complete 22 minutes of total swim time.

Week 4: Add 4 minutes to your swim time to complete 26 minutes of total swim time.

Week 5: Add 4 minutes to your swim time to complete 30 minutes of total swim time.

Session 2

Week 1: Swim for 20 minutes, 1 length fast and 1 length at recovery swim pace.

Week 2: Swim for 24 minutes, 1 length fast and 1 length at recovery swim pace.

Week 3: Swim for 20 minutes, 2 lengths fast and 1 length at recovery swim pace.

Week 4: Swim for 26 minutes, 1 length fast and 1 length at recovery pace.

Week 5: Have a fun session – try an aqua class or go to the water park and play on the slides and flumes as a celebration.

Here are some tips for when you start a swimming programme:

1. **If you are new to swimming, use a float to provide buoyancy as you kick your legs. You will still get a good cardio workout as the body has more muscle mass in the lower body than the upper body.**

2. **Swim one length 'hard' and one length 'easy' to boost the calorie-burning benefits of your swim.**

3. **Change your stokes with different lengths. For example, swim 2 lengths breaststroke to 1 length front crawl.**

4. **If you are new to exercise, intersperse water walking (see the Even Simpler Water Workout page 53) with length swimming to increase your total exercise time. Remember to try to build up to 30 minutes.**

5. **Water can be very relaxing, but if you are trying to improve your fitness and health, you will need to push yourself. To measure how hard you are working, think about your perceived rate of intensity, for you will not be able to monitor your sweat factor so well.**

So you want to get fitter?

You are up and running with your cardiovascular training and now you want to get fitter? One of the best ways to increase cardiovascular fitness is to introduce interval training. You can apply this training principle to any form of cardiovascular exercise. Running for longer, adding an extra workout session or introducing a different aerobic exercise can all create overload to help you transport oxygen around the body, but if you want to improve the oxygen consumption of your muscles, you need to start high-intensity work. This involves working at or above the anaerobic threshold (see A question of intensity, page 40). One of the most effective ways to do this is by introducing interval work into your programme.

What is interval training?

Interval training involves periods of high-intensity effort followed by recovery periods of less intense physical activity. The 30-minute Calorie-blaster Workout (page 48) is a great example of this.

Benefits of interval training

1. **You will be able to achieve more in each individual workout. Interval training increases the amount of high-intensity work you can do in a session, as you get a chance to recover in between.**
2. **You will increase the amount of calories you burn. Interval training uses mainly carbohydrate rather than fat for energy, but because of its higher intensity level it burns more calories overall.**
3. **You challenge both your aerobic and anaerobic energy systems. This provides your body with total fitness improvements.**
4. **Your training can mimic specific sports conditioning requirements. For example, let's take a game of tennis or hockey. These sports are not played at the same continuous steady pace – points get won, rallies stop and start, the ball may move from defence to attack in a short time. Interval training allows you to copy the same stop-start patterns the action will actually follow in the game, so that your body adapts specifically to the game's requirements.**
5. **You will improve your cardiovascular fitness and your body's ability to manage lactic acid.**

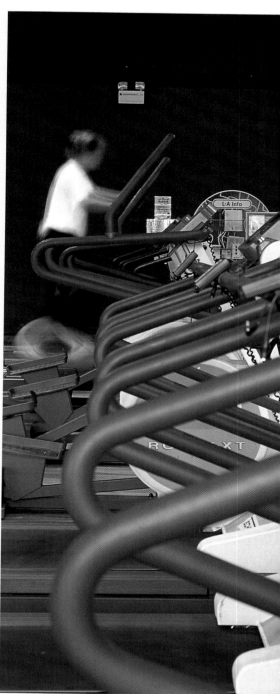

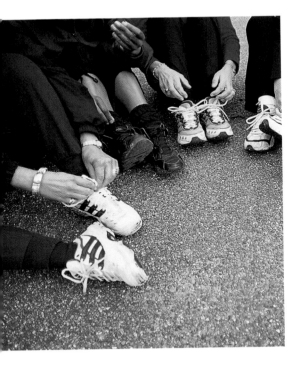

Race event preparation

Many people sign up for a long-distance event such as a half or full marathon. Raising money for charity or just the sheer physical challenge of running a marathon can be a great exercise motivator. No matter how well your training has gone, when it comes to the day, whether it's running, cycling, swimming or some other long-distance event, here are some top tips that can make your race go so much better.

Before the event

Be thoroughly prepared for the race – it's not a good time to experiment with new clothes, tactics or technique.

Practise at the same time as the start of the event. This is especially important if you have been completing most of your training in the evening after work. The event itself may be on a Sunday morning.

Do at least one shorter race during the weeks before an event. This will be of benefit because:

- **You gain valuable experience of eating and drinking on the move.**
- **You learn what it is like to complete a race at racing-pace in a crowd, how to overtake people, get drinks at water stations. Believe it or not, if you are marathon-running it is not all about just running in a straight line – you will need to do quite a bit of ducking and diving around people to ensure your own safety as well as completing an enjoyable run.**
- **You get to complete a race, which is great for your morale.**

Find out what sports drinks and foods will be available on race day and try them out on a training day – it's possible they may make you feel unwell, and if so, you don't want to wait until race day to find out. Equally, different drinks may work better for different events, and what worked for you in a running race may not be so good in a cycling event. So be prepared.

The last two days before the event…

- **Drink plenty of water.**
- **Try to get a good night's sleep both nights.**
- **Stretch your legs thoroughly a few times each day.**
- **You will have to put all your kit in an official kitbag maybe half an hour before the race, so taking a bin liner with cunningly cut arms and neck holes is a good idea. This will keep you warm and dry. Alternatively, take an old sweatshirt and a pair of tracksuit trousers that you don't mind discarding at the start of the race.**
- **Eat normally the day before (carbohydrates – especially pasta, rice, potatoes and bread – are particularly important to fuel your muscles with the essential glycogen your body will need during the event). Do not eat too much – or too little. It is unwise to 'carbo-load' unless you really know what you are doing and you have completed a long run with this nutritional technique already. Carbo-loading is not always successful for everyone.**
- **It is advisable not to drink alcohol the night before.**

Top tips for your big day

Seasoned endurance athletes often say the actual event is your victory lap. So enjoy it!

What's your name?

This is the golden rule… Print, paint, carve or scrawl your name on the FRONT of your T-shirt ABOVE the space where your race number will be. If you do this, you can be sure that, no matter how you feel, the crowd will get you around the course – but you have to help them first by letting them know who it is they are cheering for.

Sore nipples

In running events or where abrasion is likely, consider using surgical tape on your nipples to stop them rubbing against your bra or running top. It may hurt a little when you strip the tape off again, but it is not nearly as painful as jogger's nipple. Wearing a decent sports bra will also usually prevent the problem.

Don't experiment

Make sure that on race day you have the same breakfast that you have had before your long training runs. At the start of any marathon free food and drink is available, and if you are nervous you may feel tempted. However, as I know from personal experience, it's wisest to eat only what you are used to eating just before a run – otherwise you could regret it later.

Grease-up

Use petroleum jelly to grease your toes, inside thighs and anywhere else you think has even the faintest chance of chafing.

Wear gloves

If the weather is cold, forget your street credibility and consider taking a pair of lightweight gloves.

Zipped and fastened

Ensure your clothes are properly and comfortably fastened before you start the race – it is very difficult to adjust your clothing or tie your laces if you have, say, 30,000 runners, as in the London Marathon, stampeding after you.

Saddlebags

You may have taken up long-distance events to get rid of your 'saddle-bags', but wearing a sports bum bag can be a useful way to carry sports nutrition bars or gels. If you are planning to take your own sports drink in a bottle, make sure it does not leak.

During the race

- **Do not start off too fast. Psychologically it is harder to keep going if you are constantly being overtaken, but easier if you have enough energy to overtake others later on.**
- **Keep an even pace throughout – if you really want to sprint and you feel up to it, wait until the last 3m/3yd. If you suddenly collapse, the momentum will still get you over the line.**
- **Make sure you have taken on enough water before the start – hoping that you can make up a water-deficit during a race is pure wishful thinking. If you have not drunk enough before the race, it is too late. Dehydration will impair your performance drastically.**
- **Take on water regularly – i.e. at most, if not all, drinks stations, which are situated**

every 1.6km/1mile. You should aim to take on at least 0.5 litres/1 pint an hour or three or more gulps at every station. If it's a hot day, take on more. Do not drink from the refreshing sponges which are given out sporadically – they're often full of chemicals.
- **If injured as opposed to just plain shattered – stop running. You may still be able to complete the event walking if the pain is not too great.**
- **Try to go with the flow. Remember, if you have not done a marathon before, you are aiming to complete a finishing time – not a winning time.**

After the race

- **Golden Rule: DRINK LOADS OF WATER.**
- **Even though you are tired, put your warm, dry kit on as soon as possible.**
- **Try to stretch properly (this may be easier said than done).**
- **Do not plan on having to walk too far after the finish to go anywhere – you may not feel like it.**
- **Eat a meal high in carbohydrates within 2 hours of finishing the event. It will help you replenish your lost muscle glycogen.**
- **Be prepared for muscle soreness – walking up stairs may feel okay, but walking down stairs will most definitely be painful, as a result of the eccentric muscle work you have done.**
- **During the week after the event, keep your training very light – and give yourself a couple of days' rest first.**

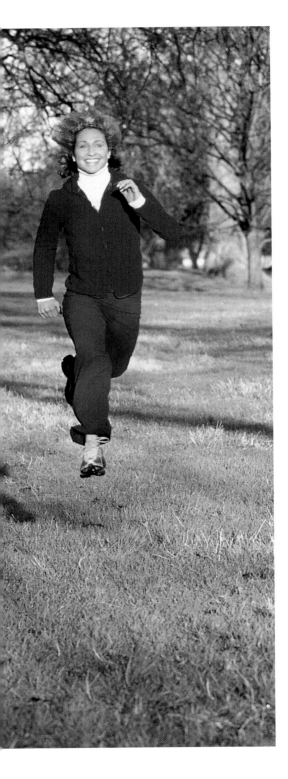

Questions and answers

Q Help! I can't run! How do I start?

A Starting to run can be a little daunting – and it is not a good idea to go out and just try to run as far as you can straight away. You will increase your risk of injury, may well feel nauseous and find the experience extremely unpleasant. You will probably give up and resolve never to go through that pain again. So if you want to learn how to run, here is a 12-week plan to get your legs moving, your heart pumping and those feel-good endorphins buzzing. Perform each training session 3 times a week. You can do it on a treadmill at the gym or outside in the park – it really is that simple. Once you have done that, you can progress to the Beginner's Jogging Programme on page 45.

Here's what you do:

Weeks 1–2	Run 30 seconds, walk 90 seconds x 10
Weeks 3–4	Run 60 seconds, walk 60 seconds x 10
Weeks 5–6	Run 90 seconds, walk 90 seconds x 7
Weeks 7–8	Run 2 mins, walk 1 min x 7
Weeks 9–10	Run 3 mins, walk 1 min x 5
Weeks 11–12	Run 4 mins, walk 1 min x 4

Q I would really like to cycle more quickly. My partner and children always seem to be so much further ahead of me when we go for rides at the weekend.

A We need to work towards increasing the intensity of your cycling. You may be putting in the time in the saddle, but if you are always cycling at the same pace your body will not get fitter and you will not be able to increase your speed. So here is a simple 30-minute interval workout to increase your speed and burn those tyres!

Intensity level
10 seconds hard/10 seconds easy x 10
Recover for 3 mins
Repeat x 5

Q I have just started jogging – I enjoy going out every weekend, but I get a little embarrassed as I am always getting overtaken in the park by other runners. I know I should not be worried, but it would just be nice to be overtaking them for a change and not the other way round!

A You need to work on the cardiovascular stamina of your legs, heart and lungs. As you get fitter, your leg muscles are able to extract and use more oxygen from your blood supply. Here is a simple 20-minute treadmill workout that will help you increase your speed. Add this to your existing running programme, achieving a total of 4 workouts a week.

Run 3 mins at speed A
Run harder for 1 min (increase speed)
Run 3 mins at speed A
Run harder 1 min (increase speed again)
Run 3 mins at speed A
Run harder for 1 min (increase speed again)
Run 3 mins at speed A
Run harder for 1 min (increase speed again)
Run 3 mins at speed A
Run harder for 1 min (increase speed again)

Q I want to get fit for squash. I really like the game, but I get out of breath so quickly.

A You need to build up your cardio base first. This will strengthen your heart and lungs and help your body supply energy to the working muscles more effectively. (See Body laid bare, page 39). So first complete the 'I can't run. How do I start'? Programme and then follow it with the rope-skipping interval programme (below), which mimics the stop-start nature of your game.

Warm-up
Run/power-walk 4 mins
60 seconds rope-skipping
Run/power-walk 4 mins
60 seconds rope-skipping
Run/power-walk 4 mins
60 seconds rope-skipping
Run/power-walk 4 mins
60 seconds rope-skipping
Run/power-walk 4 mins
60 seconds rope-skipping
Run/power-walk 4 mins
60 seconds rope-skipping
Run/power-walk 4 mins
Cool Down

Q I have entered a 5km/3.1 mile fun run. As a mum, working shifts, I don't have a lot of time to put into my training, but this will be my second event, so I would really like to improve on my time. What should I do?

A Good for you – it's great to have a goal to work towards. It will keep you focused, for you can't move your goal – so here is a planning suggestion. It's time-efficient and results-orientated.

Weeks 1–2	Run hard for 200m/run easy for 200m x 8
Weeks 3–4	Run hard for 200m/run easy for 200m x 9
Weeks 5–6	Run hard for 200m/run easy for 200m x 10
Weeks 7–8	Run hard for 200m/run easy for 200m x 11
Weeks 9–10	Run hard for 200m/run easy for 200m x 12

Q I want to improve on my half-marathon running time. I have a place in the London Marathon and as part of my training I have read that it is a good idea to do a half-marathon. I have done one before, but I was very slow – it took me 3 hours. How can I achieve a better time?

A Never be embarrassed about your first running time – any first event can be nerve-racking. You have learnt from the experience, and now is the time to put in some training so that you can enjoy your half-marathon and be fully prepared for your full marathon. When planning your overall race preparation, you may wish to schedule in a half-marathon and a longer-distance event, such as 30km/18$\frac{1}{2}$ miles. This will give you as much race practice as possible.

Weeks 1–2	On weekly long run, run half the distance at a slow pace, run back 2 mins faster.
Weeks 3–4	Run half the distance at a slow pace, run back 4 mins faster.
Weeks 5–6	Run half the distance at a slow pace, run back 6 mins faster.
Weeks 7–8	Run half the distance at a slow pace, run back 7 mins faster.
Weeks 9–10	Run half the distance at a slow pace, run back 8 mins faster.
Weeks 11–12	Run half the distance at a slow pace, run back 9 mins faster.

Q Help! I have so little time! What can I do?

A This is such a common problem. We are all faced with the challenge of not having enough time to exercise, but don't panic! I have devised three short workouts – one for the gym, one to do at home (see page 47). And, when you're REALLY short of time, just remember that simply moving more often is the foundation to overall health, so take a look at the pedometer walking step targets (see page 38) and aim for a minimum of 4,000 steps a day. These can be accumulated right through the day, while you go about your daily activities. You'll find you get in more excercise, though, if you leave your mobile and the TV remote in another room – and if you start to park your car on the other side of the car park!

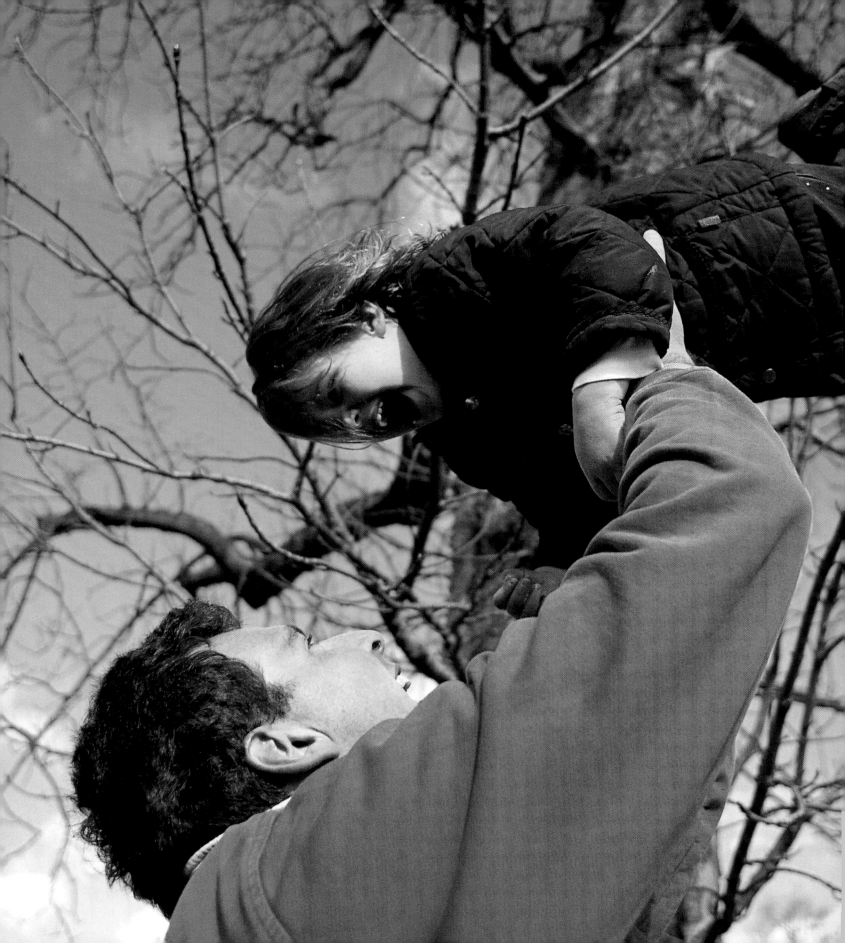

resistance exercise

Only a decade ago exercise prescription typically consisted of cardiovascular activity and the odd leg stretch. Little or no emphasis was given to resistance training, especially for women. Today all this has changed, and resistance training is popular with men and women. Effective resistance training develops a toned and shapely body, improved power and strength, and enhanced sports performance. But resistance training also provides important health benefits such as stronger bones, reduced susceptibility to injury and reduced risk of osteoporosis.

And if you still have lingering doubts, read on. Yes, resistance training does involve working with some kind of weight, but if you do the exercises as described in this chapter, you will not end up with big bulky muscles bulging out of your workout top. Instead you will see and feel real improvements in your body shape and self-esteem.

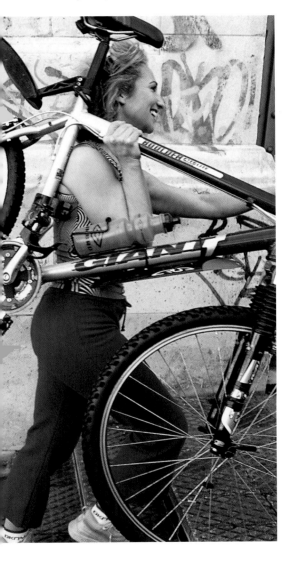

What is resistance exercise?

Resistance exercise involves exerting a force to enable you to move or apply tension to a weight, and results in enhanced muscular strength and endurance. The intensity and repetition with which the force is applied determine whether the exercise is building up muscular endurance or muscular strength.

Muscular *endurance* is a measure of the number of times a muscle can repeat a contraction, whereas muscular *strength* relates to the force a muscle can apply in a contraction. Clearly muscular endurance has a significant part to play in our everyday life: consider the number of times we need to pick up our children, carry the shopping, etc. But muscular strength has an important role too.

As we grow older, our strength slowly declines, but somewhere around the age of 55 it starts to decline more rapidly because we lose essential muscle protein. What we may have considered a relatively easy task may now require full muscular strength. Think of an elderly person who finds it hard to get up out of an armchair unassisted. The difficulty they experience is caused by the lack of

muscular strength in their quadriceps, hamstrings and gluteals. So if you intend to stay physically active and independent beyond your 50th birthday, you should add some sort of resistance exercise to your activity programme.

To improve both muscular strength and muscular endurance, the body needs to be trained in different ways. To increase your muscular endurance, you need to build up the number of repetitive contractions the targeted muscle or part of the body can do under a point of tension. Endurance training involves low resistance with high repetitions.

Just as your cardiovascular system needs to be pushed to a point of overload for the heart to get stronger and more efficient, so you need to overload the muscles each time you train (see pages 16 and 40 so that you get to the point of near-fatigue. In resistance training, this is when you feel your muscle can perform only one or two more lifts with good technique. Near-fatigue represents that point at which the muscle has or is just about to reach the point of overload. Helping your body to reach that point of near-fatigue is not just about adding more weight. Simple ways to challenge the body include performing more repetitions, increasing the number of workouts or sets of repetitions per week, holding the length of lift for longer, and changing the order of your exercises.

These all challenge the body, and its response will be to get stronger and more toned.

Over a training period, effective overload with muscular endurance training benefits the muscles in several ways. Your body will increase:

- **the number of aerobic enzymes and mitochondria**
- **the density of blood capillaries**
- **the efficiency of muscular contractions**

As a muscle is required to repeat its contractions a number of times, these adaptations are similar to the aerobic adaptations we see with cardiovascular training. The changes encourage the delivery of more oxygen to the working muscle and improve its ability to convert it to energy. The end result is that it becomes easier for you to lift the weight repeatedly.

Increased strength comes about through lifting heavy loads a few times. Strength training uses high resistance with fewer repetitions, and with effective overload your body will experience the following adaptations:

- **More contractile protein**
- **Tougher connective tissue**
- **Increased muscular contractibility**

During strength training, the aerobic capacity of the muscle is not so challenged; instead, the muscle is stimulated to get stronger so that it can lift more weight, exerting more force against the bone, and overcome greater resistances. Strength training may mean

Body laid bare
And now for the science bit….

When a muscle contracts, crossbridges in the muscle fibres known as actin and myosin draw closer together, creating the necessary tension to overcome the force. During a contraction, muscles can either shorten, lengthen or stay the same. Muscle contractions that involve the muscle getting shorter are called concentric contractions, and occur with a lifting action. For example, you contract your bicep muscles concentrically when you lift a dumbbell.

Muscle contractions that involve the muscle lengthening are called eccentric. These muscles are put under tension as a force is lowered or returned to a position with control. Think about a drawbridge lowering across a moat: if there were no controlling tension, the bridge would come crashing down. It's a similar thing with eccentric muscle contractions. When you lower your dumbbell from your biceps curl, your muscles are contracting eccentrically.

Isometric contractions occur when your muscles are under tension but there is no movement at the joint. Lifting your dumbbell and holding the position half-way through the movement would be an isometric contraction of the biceps. We use all these types of contractions in everyday life. With your resistance training programmes, however, it is better to work the muscles through their full range of motion using concentric and eccentric contractions. Isometric contractions can have more of a specific sports application.

the muscle becomes larger, as more contractile proteins are laid down in each muscle fibre. This is known as hypertrophy.

For the average female these increases can be quite small, as she has less testosterone – a hormone associated with muscle mass – than the average male. The improvements in a woman's strength are more to do with increased co-ordination and ability to

recruit the correct muscle fibres together.

Not all muscles are created equal. Simply speaking, there are two main types of contracting muscles: slow-twitch and fast-twitch. Each has specific properties, which make them more suited to particular activities. Slow-twitch fibres are designed for more continuously, aerobic activity. They have a greater supply of aerobic enzymes and a denser blood capillary network. Fast-twitch fibres are

Strength training benefits

1. **Improved strength and power.** Improvements in strength and power have a direct impact on the quality of our day-to-day living. Studies have shown that women who undertake strength training are able to walk more quickly and for longer.

2. **Increased bone strength.** Improvements in bone density reduce the incidence of osteoporosis. And the sooner you start bone loading, the greater the protective effect.

3. **Increased lean body mass.** An increased lean muscle mass will boost your metabolic rate. This means you will be burning more calories in your sleep.

4. **Increased functional fitness.** Everyday activities can be performed with greater ease.

5. **Improved glucose tolerance.** Studies have shown that decreased abdominal obesity, brought about by strength training, improves glucose intolerance, reducing the risk of late-onset diabetes.

6. **Improved balance and walking gait.** Increased muscle strength around the hip and knee joints improves balance and reduces the risk of falls.

better designed for shorter, more intense, activities such as resistance work. Fast-twitch muscle fibres respond more favourably to strength training, as they have greater anaerobic energy capacities necessary for this kind of training. Muscular strength training increases the cross-sectional diameter of each muscle fibre, providing more protein filaments and cross-bridges in the muscle to apply force. This is in part explains why strength training can increase the size of the muscle while muscular endurance training can create more toning effects.

A question of intensity

Just as different levels of intensity in your cardiovascular work result in different adaptations to your body, so too do different resistance intensities.

For novice strength exercisers:

1–3 sets of 10–12 repetitions are recommended. After the first 2 weeks, exercisers can advance to 3 sets of 10–12 repetitions and increase your chosen starting weight by 900g–2.25kg/2–5lb. Most weight-training workouts are performed 2–3 times per week on alternate days; for example, Monday and Wednesday, or Monday, Wednesday and Friday. For further variety check out the different weight equipment available on page 66

For more advanced lifters:

For advanced lifters who are working towards a strength, rather than an endurance, objective, anywhere from 3 to 15 repetitions are recommended, depending on the specific aims of the weight-training programme. In addition, more frequent weight-training workouts can be conducted, exercising alternate muscle groups on different days (for instance,. strength training for the lower body on Monday and Wednesday, and upper-body exercises on Tuesday and Thursday).

How little can I get away with?

For general health and fitness purposes, the most widely recognized prescription for strength training comes from the American College of Sports Medicine and the United States Surgeon General. They recommend a single set of 8–12 repetitions 3 or more times a week. Although single sets of resistance exercises have generally been regarded as beginners' fare, there is growing evidence that single-set workouts can provide similar benefits to a 3-set regimen. In fact, studies have shown significant improvements in muscular strength, muscular endurance and body composition with single-set workouts compared with multiple workouts. While multiple sets may produce greater muscular endurance improvements, if you are short on time but still demand results you can achieve the results you want through single-set workouts. So if you are a time-conscious exerciser who seeks muscular fitness improvements, single-set training programmes can be an effective option. (You will find that some of the workouts in *The exercise bible* require 2 or 3 sets. These have been specifically designed for optimum results, but you will still benefit from a single set.)

To increase strength:

To see an improvement in your physical strength, fewer repetitions at higher resistances are recommended. Rest intervals between sets should be long enough so that maximum loads can be lifted (this is roughly equivalent to 90 seconds).

To optimize gains in muscle endurance, and for muscle toning:

- Use lower weights with more repetitions.
- But remember: the key to any resistance-training programme is the ability to sustain it, and you still need to reach that point of near-fatigue, whether you are looking to improve endurance or strength.

Getting started

Resistance-training workouts should contain a general warm-up and a more body-specific warm-up. The warm-up should include activities that use the whole body, such as brisk walking, jogging, stationary cycling and stretching.

A more specific warm-up should include exercises that will be performed in the main workout section but with a lighter weight or smaller range of motion. These specific exercises prepare the muscle for the joint motions required. At the end of each workout, remember to stretch the main muscle used. See page 129–135, for specific muscle stretches.

Designing a resistance programme

When you design a resistance programme, it is important to adopt a whole-body approach to your training, using all your major muscle groups. Take into account the following:

1. **Go for symmetry.**
   Remember to work both sides of the body. For example – work the abdominals and strengthen your back muscles.
2. **Variety of movement.**
   Select different exercises and different joint actions to get a more balanced programme.

3. **Change the exercises every 6–8 weeks.**
   This will stop you getting bored, help you avoid over-use injuries and muscular imbalances and keep your muscles guessing – all necessary if you want to improve your shape, tone and strength.
4. **Add extra intensity each 4th workout.**
   This is an easy way to overload your muscles progressively. Slow the exercise down, add more weight, add extra repetitions or an extra set, or work through the lifting phase more than the lowering phase.
5. **Avoid rushing.**
   Complete your movements smoothly and slowly. Do not rush each exercise and focus on your technique as you complete each movement. Different muscles have different points of weakness so try to execute each contraction with control, avoiding jerky actions, through the whole range of the motion.

Equipment

Traditionally we think of weights as the free weights or the fixed-weight equipment we find in the gym. However, when we train to improve our muscular endurance and strength, our muscles do not know whether they are lifting a 4.5kg/10lb box of groceries or a 4.5kg/10lb barbell. Anything can provide the muscles with a strength impetus. Tubing and resistance bands, hand weights, water bottles, medicine balls, fixed weights, even body weight, can all provide the required strength stimulus if used in the correct way.

The following table lists the pros and cons of the different types of weights.

	PLUS POINTS	MINUS POINTS
Weight machines (e.g. Smith machine, lateral pull-down)	• Safe • Easy to use • Work all the major muscle groups • Minimal skill required, so good for new exerciser	• High cost • Limited number of exercises • Body restricted to move only in way body is positioned • Bulky, requiring space
Free weights (e.g. barbell, body bar)	• A wide variety of different exercises are possible • Allow mimicry of true movement • Cheaper to buy than fixed weights • More easily stored than fixed weights	• Require greater skill from exerciser – body not pre-positioned, so novice exerciser at greater risk of injury • Require training partner to ensure good technique and help with positioning
Tubing or resistance bands	• Cheap • Easy to store • Portable • Different strengths of tubing available to create overload • Allows work through different joint angles and therefore may reduce risk of injury caused by overuse	• Correct positioning of body required to ensure good results and technique • Can cause chafing of skin if tubing held against bare legs – this can be especially uncomfortable if you have body hair • If you are very strong, tubing may not be able to provide enough load
Own body weight	• Costs you nothing • Goes with you everywhere! • Positioning your body cleverly against gravity can create effective overload	• Some muscle groups are not challenged effectively – e.g. biceps and deltoids require external resistance

Best Body Bits

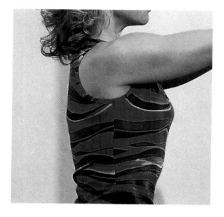
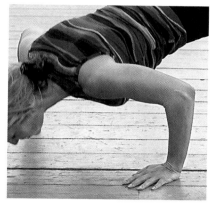
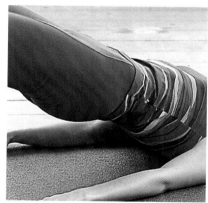
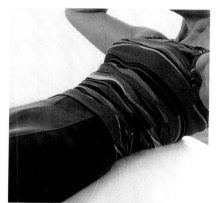
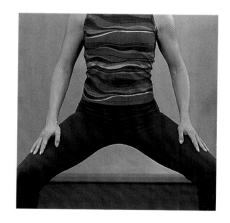
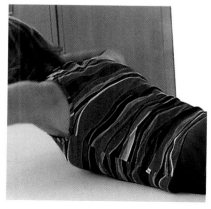

We all have a part of the body we'd like to improve, and, if we're lucky, a bit we're proud of and want to enhance even more. In this section you'll find top, simple-to-follow exercises specifically designed to improve individual parts of your body. For each body bit I've devised essential exercises to improve the tone, shape and balance of that muscle group. Do the exercises 3 times a week for 4 weeks and you will definitely see and feel a difference. You will find the number of repetitions you need to do beside each exercise, but remember that as you get fitter you will need to do more, and with heavier weights, depending on your training aims. Remember: lower repetitions and greater weight stimulate strength gains, while lower weight with more repetitions will create toning effects. Oh, and don't forget you do not need to reach that point of near-fatigue! (See page 62 for more information.)

Chest

Body Kit

Bench

Hand weights

Smith machine

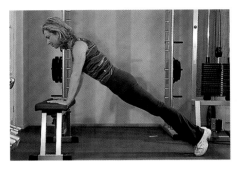 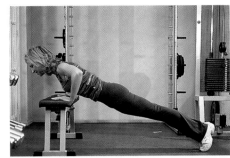

Inclined Press-up

What it does: Strengthens and tones chest pectoral muscles.

What you do: Position your hands more than shoulder-distance apart on a bench. Step back so your body is inclined in a straight line from your feet to your shoulders. Make sure your abdominals are contracted and your shoulder blades are down. Focus on keeping the neck long to help you achieve this. Slowly bend the elbows lowering the chest towards the bench, and press back up to the straight-arm position.

How many? 12–16

Top Tip: The higher the bench, the easier this exercise is.

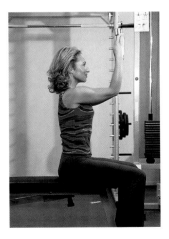 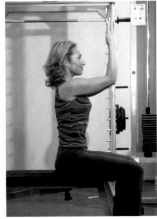

Elbow Bust Press

What it does: Specifically targets the inner muscle fibres of the chest pectoral muscles, helping to draw the bust together.

What you do: Sit with good posture, feet flat on the floor under the knees. Lift the arms so the elbows are bent at 90° to the shoulder. Press the elbows, forearms and hands together. Keeping the elbows high, lift the hands up towards the ceiling. Keep the forearms pressed together. Slowly lower the elbows back to the start position. NB Keep the elbows high – allowing them to drop will reduce the effectiveness of this exercise.

How many? 12–16

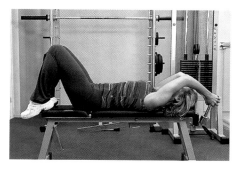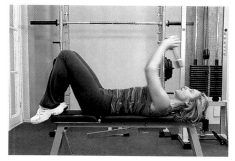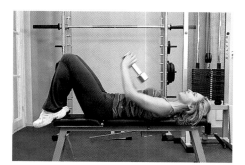

Pullover

What it does: Targets the upper fibres of the chest pectoral muscles to support and lift the bust line.

What you do: Lie on your back with your spine in neutral position. Hold a 2.25–4.5kg/5–10lb weight in both hands above the head-line. Keeping the elbows bent and shoulder-distance apart, draw the weight in over the head and lower in a controlled manner to the belly button. Slowly lift the weight back over the head again. Focus on keeping the ribs and hips connected in this position.

How many? 12–16

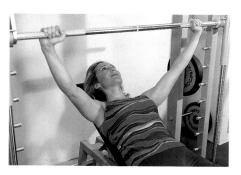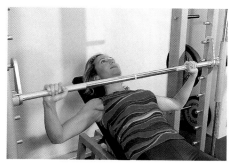

Inclined Bench Press

What it does: Targets the whole of the chest pectoral muscle as well as the deltoids.

What you do: Lie on an inclined bench, and using a Smith machine (see page 66) hold the bar across the nipple-line of the body and press up, extending the arms straight. Slowly lower the weight down towards the chest with the arms wide.

How many? 12–16

Top Tip: If you do not have a Smith machine in your gym, you can use a body bar or free weights instead.

Arms

Body Kit

Foam roll

Small hand weights

Resistance band/tubing

Exercise ball

Chair

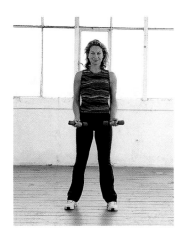

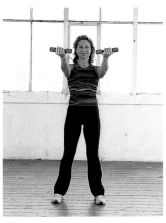

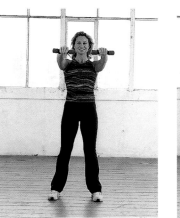

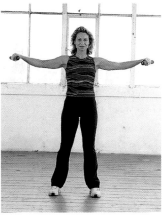

Two-way Shoulder Raise

What it does: Creates definition in shoulders.

What you do: Stand with feet hip-distance apart, a 2.25–4.5kg/5–10lb weight in each hand. Lift the arms forwards to shoulder height with palms facing up. Bend the elbows slightly and take the arms sideways at shoulder height, then lower them to the side.

How many? 12–16 reps.

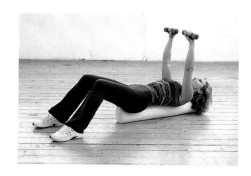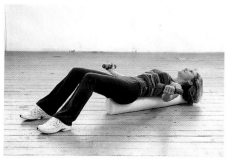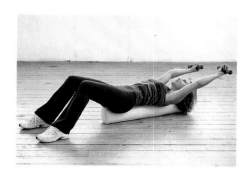

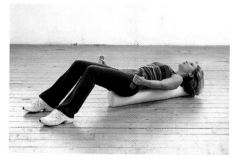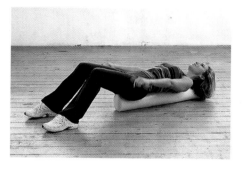

Prone Full Arm Circle

What it does: Tones the front and back of the the arm.

What you do: Lie face-up with the spine in neutral position (see illustration on page 78). Start with the arms overhead and a small weight in each hand. Slowly lower the arms above the head, opening them to the side as if they are drawing a circle. Keep the elbows soft and shoulder blades down. Keep the hands off the floor. Repeat the other way.

How many? 8–10 in each direction

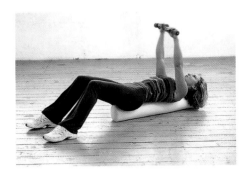
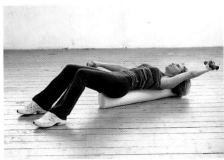
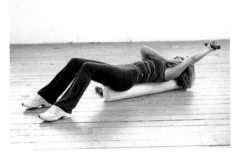

Scissors

What it does: Tones the backs of the arms and gives the arms lean definition.

What you do: Lie on your back, arms extended directly over the eye-line. Hold one small weight (about 900g–1.35kg/2–3lb) in each hand. Lower the arms in opposite directions, one over your head, the other down to your thighs. Keep the weight off the floor, lengthen through the arm as you lower, and keep the wrist in neutral position. Draw the arms back overhead and scissor in the other direction.

How many? Take 4 counts to complete this move. Hold out and raise one hand 7.5cm/3in off the floor and then repeat on the other side. Perform 12 repetitions on each arm.

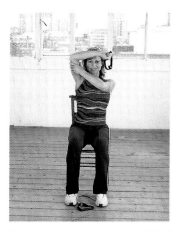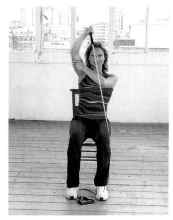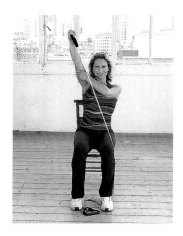

Triceps Extension With Resistance Band

What it does: Tones the backs of the arms.

What you do: Start seated with one hand in front of you holding the tubing and the other hand above your head, with your elbow bent to the side. Extend the arm straight, rotating the hand out to the side. Control the arm back down.

How many? 12–16

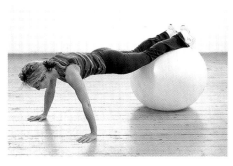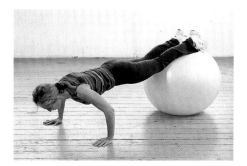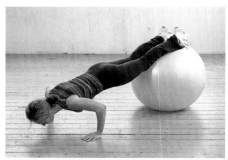

Declined Wide Arm Press-up

What it does: Tones the shoulders and the backs of the arms.

What you do: Start with your knees and lower legs on an exercise ball, hands on the floor and arms straight in line with your shoulders. Keep your body straight from head to tailbone. Bend your elbows, lowering the torso until the elbows are about in line with the shoulders. Push up.

How many: 12–16

Buttocks

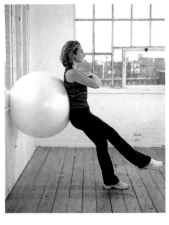 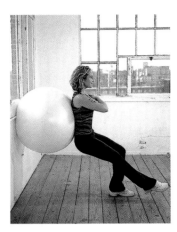

One-leg Ball Squat

What it does: Tightens the gluteus muscle.

What you do: Put an exercise ball against a wall and stand with your lower back firmly and comfortably against it. Cross your arms over your chest, hands over opposite shoulders. Walk your feet forwards about one stride's length, feet hip-distance apart. Step your left foot in front of the centre of the ball and lift your right foot. With abdominals contracted, chest lifted and lower back in neutral position, bend the knee to roll the ball down the wall. Lower the hips, thighs parallel and balance with your foot flat on the ground. Pressing through your heel, drive the hips back up as you straighten your working leg.

How many? 10–12 on each leg

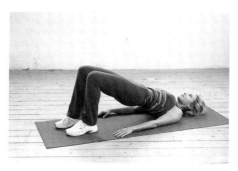 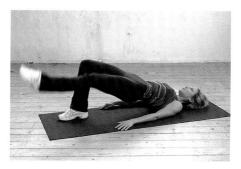 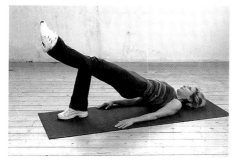

Bridge With Leg Lift

What it does: Tightens the gluteus muscle.

What you do: Lie on your back, knees bent, feet flat on the floor, arms at your side. From a neutral pelvis position use the hips, thigh and trunk muscles to lift the pelvis off the floor until the body forms one line from your shoulders to your knees. Extend one leg straight, lift it level with the knee and lower to the floor.

How many? 10 on each leg

Top Tip: Keep the hips level with a deep contraction in the supporting leg's buttocks.

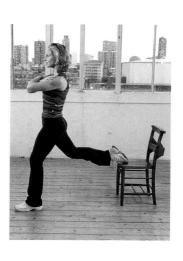 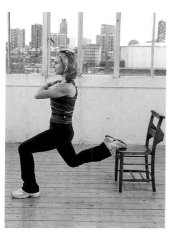

Reverse Lunge

What it does: Lifts the buttock cheeks up from the top of the thighs.

What you do: Stand a stride-length away in front of a bench or chair with your feet hip-distance apart. Hold a dumbbell in each hand at your sides. If you're not using weights, rest your hands across your chest. Place your right foot on top of the bench. Keep the chest lifted, abdominal muscles tight and back erect, bend your knees and lower your hips towards the floor. Make sure you keep the right knee over the right ankle and in line with the second toe. Use your buttocks to drive your hips back up to the starting position. Finish the set and repeat on the other side. If new to this exercise, start with a low bench and progress to a higher one.

How many? 12–16 on each leg

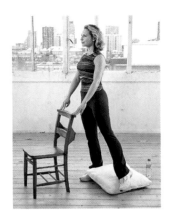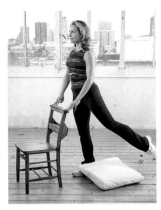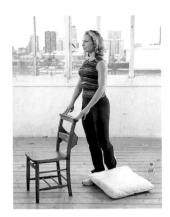

Standing Leg Circle

What it does: Lifts and draws the buttocks together.

What you do: Place a cushion and water bottle on the floor. Stand with feet cushion-width apart. Extend one leg with the toe resting on the outside of the cushion and lengthen through the leg. If you wish, hold on to a chair for balance, as you draw a circle with the leg over the cushion and water bottle. Bring the foot of the working leg to rest behind the supporting leg's ankle. Keep the knee turned out and lift the working leg directly back behind the supporting leg. Lower down, and draw a circle with the leg back over the cushion and water bottle to return to the start position.

How many? 16–20 on each leg

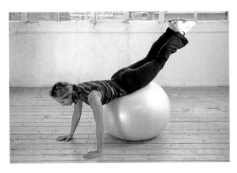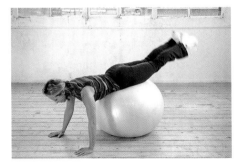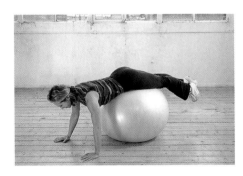

Prone Ball Hip Extension

What it does: Lifts the buttock area.

What you do: Drape your body over the exercise ball and place your hands on the floor in front of you with your legs separated. The ball should be sized so that it fits in the crease of your hips. With the abdominals tight and lower back supported, use the gluteal muscles to lift both legs up and together until they are in line with the rest of the torso. Bending like a hinge from the hips, return to a starting position. For an easier version, lift one leg at a time.

How many? 16–20

Top Tip: You may be lying on your belly but make sure you keep your abdominals contracted to support your spine.

Abdominals

Body Kit
Towel
Exercise ball
Broom handle or pole
Tennis ball

A word about technique

Abdominal exercises are often among the most poorly executed. We all want a flat abdominal area – but sometimes doing more exercise does not mean you get better results. Here are some top tips to help you really get that flat belly.

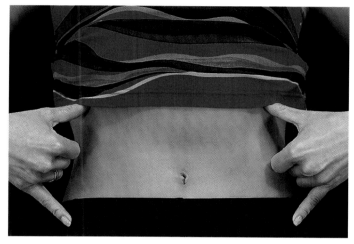

The Rib–hip Connection

When you lie on the floor before you start, make sure you have a connection between your ribs and your hips. This will help you contract the abdominals before you lift and ensure you are in the correct anatomical position for your spine. Here is what you do. Place your thumb on your bottom ribs and your fingers on the top of the hip bone. Draw these two points together with a small contraction of the abdominal muscles. Your spine should be in a neutral position. This neutral position will vary from person to person depending on the shape of the spine. However, there should be a small space between the floor and your back. Keep the rib–hip connection so you maintain your neutral position to establish trunk stability.

One you have masered this technique, you will really start to see an improvement in your abdominal training.

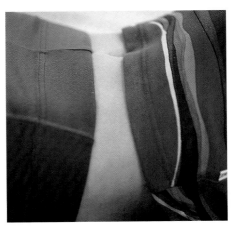

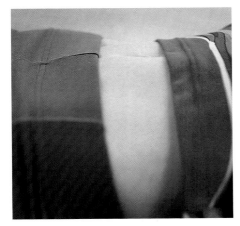

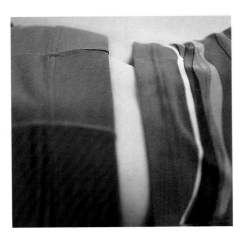

Common mistakes

- **Problem: Pressing your back too far into the floor.**

  It makes the hip flexor muscle contract excessively and can put additional strain on the back, causing muscle imbalance.

  Solution: Redo your rib–hip connection to check you are in the right position, and focus on keeping your tail bone down on the floor.

- **Problem: Arching your back off the floor.**

  This will cause your abdominal muscles to pull on the lower spine as you perform your abdominal work.

  Solution: Redo your rib–hip connection and make sure that you rest when you start to feel tired in your abdominals. Performing the exercises with poor technique can often result in the back arching.

- **Correct position.**

  You have established rib-hip connection contracting your abdominals to create a neutral position and support for your spine.

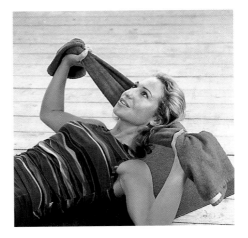

Neck support

Many people complain of feeling pain in the neck when starting abdominal work. This is quite common and generally relates to the fact that the abdominals are weak and the neck muscles are helping to lift the body up.

Solution: Take a towel and place it behind the head. Hold both ends taut so it supports the neck. Keep the towel taut as you curl up and down.

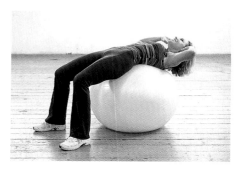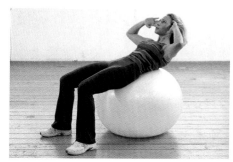

Ball Crunch

What it does: Tones the upper abdominal muscles.

What you do: Sit on an exercise ball, feet flat on the floor. Cross the arms over the chest. Establish trunk stability and walk the feet out so the knees are aligned with the ankles. Curl the head, neck and shoulders up until the shoulder blades clear the ball and the pelvis is lifted forward. Lower and repeat.

How many? 16–20. Perform a second set after a 45-second rest if necessary, to create overload

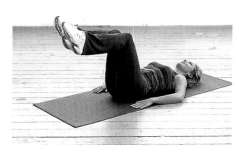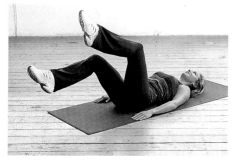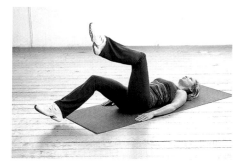

Toe Touch

What it does: Flattens the lower abdominal wall, especially the transverse muscle.

What you do: Lie on your back with knees over hips and feet parallel to floor. Establish trunk stability. Slowly lower one leg down, dropping the heel to the floor. Keep the spine in neutral position as you lift the leg back over the chest. Repeat on the other side. The trick with this exercise is to perform it slowly and focus on form. To make the exercise easier, bend the leg more and lower it to the floor closer to your bottom.

How many? Build up to 16 on each leg

Top Tip: This is a challenging exercise. Start out trying to do a few repetitions with really good technique.

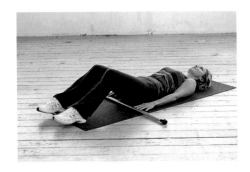
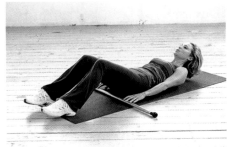
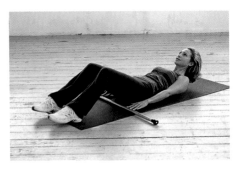
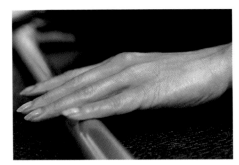

Abdominal Curl With Bar Roll

What it does: Tightens the upper abdominals, especially around the rib area. This is especially good post-pregnancy when the rib cage has often extended to allow room for the growing baby.

What you do: Lie on floor, knees bent. Place a body bar, broom handle or pole on the floor between your feet and bottom, and slide the feet away from your bottom until you feel the toes start to come off the floor. Establish trunk tension and rest your fingers lightly on the bar. Keeping your fingers on the bar, slowly push it towards your toes as you curl around your rib cage. Draw the ribs down towards the pelvis as you lift. To do this, imagine you are wearing a corset and you are trying to keep the rib cage small.

How many? 16–20

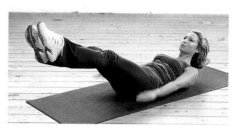 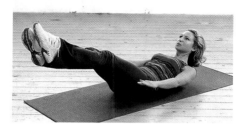

'Hundreds'

What it does: This is a Pilates exercise which flattens the whole of the abdominal area.

What you do: Lie on the floor, face up. Establish trunk tension with a neutral spine. Lift the legs off the floor, extending them away from your body. Curl the upper body off the floor. Keep this contracted abdominal position as you beat your arms to the floor.

How many? Breathe out for 5 beats and breathe in for 5 beats. Repeat until you have counted to 100.

Top Tip: Ensure the abdominals are connected throughout this exercise (see The Rib-hip Connection, page 77). Take a rest if you need to. For an easier version keep your feet flat on the floor.

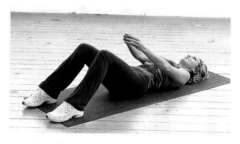 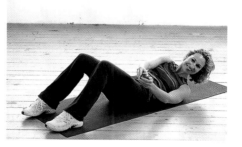 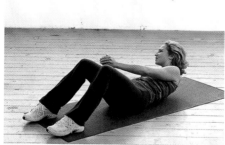

Ball Offering

What it does: Tightens the waist area. Using the ball helps to contract the oblique muscles more and prevent tension in the neck.

What you do: Lie on your back, face-up, with a neutral spine. Hold a small ball in both hands. Slowly curl to the outer side of each calf. Keep the shoulders relaxed and draw in through the navel as you rotate. Focus on drawing the bottom right rib closer to the opposite left hip, and ensure you keep some trunk tension as you uncurl. To avoid rolling the lower body as you rotate, place a small ball between your knees and keep the same tension on the ball as you rotate.

How many? 16–20 on each side

Thighs

Body Kit

Your body!

Step

Mat

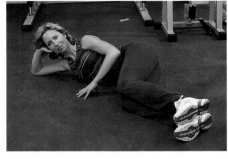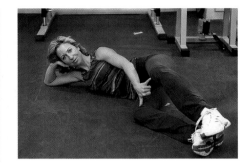

Can Opener

What it does: Tones the outer thigh.

What you do: Lie on your side, legs at 90° to your chest and knees 90° to your feet. As you look down towards your knees, you should just be able to see your toes. Keep the inner part of the feet together and open your thighs, hinging at the hips and the feet. Try to open the knees as far apart as possible. Slowly lower in a controlled manner. Make sure your hips stay stacked and your abdominals contracted.

How many? 12 slow with 8 small lifts at the widest point of the movement

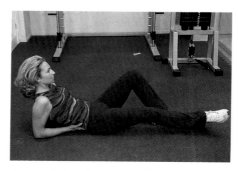 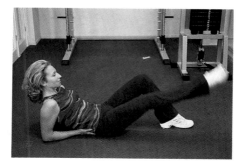 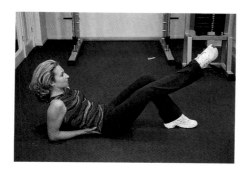

Inner Thigh Leg Lift

What it does: Streamlines inner adductor muscle.

What you do: Lie on your back, supporting yourself on your elbows. Extend one leg straight and bend the other at the knee with the foot flat on the floor. Rotate the straight leg at the hip so the inner thigh is turned to the sky. Imagine you are stretching the straight leg as long as possible, but keep a slight bend at the knee (often referred to as a 'soft knee').

How many? 12–16

Top Tip: Keep the foot relaxed – this helps you target the inner thigh more.

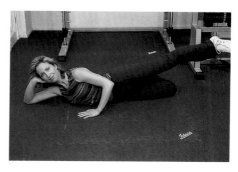 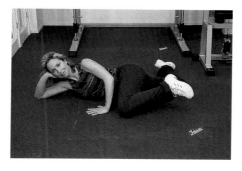 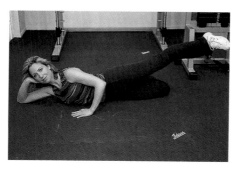

Single Leg Press

What it does: Tones the outer thighs and tightens the outer buttock muscles.

What you do: Lie on your side, bottom leg bent, with hip, knee and upper body forming one line. Your top arm will provide some support for your body. Extend your top leg to about a 40° angle, with the foot relaxed and toe slightly turned down. Stabilizing the abdominals, draw the knee into the hand on the floor and extend the leg diagonally away down the length of the body. Ensure your abdominals are contracted so that the pelvis remains stabilized throughout the exercise.

How many? 16

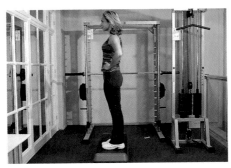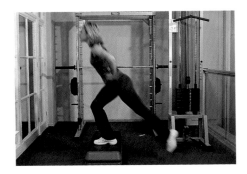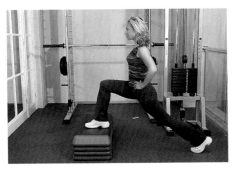

Straight Leg Lunge

What it does: Tones the quadriceps, hamstrings, buttocks and calves.

What you do: Stand on a step, maintaining good posture. Taking a large stride off the step, extending one leg back. The front knee should be over the front ankle and the back leg should be long with a slight bend at the knee. Keep the back knee and heel off the floor. Contract through the abdominals as you lift yourself back up to a straight position. Change legs.

How many? 12 on each leg

Top Tip: To help with your balance, contract up through the pelvic floor muscles as you lift.

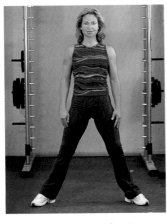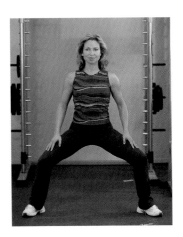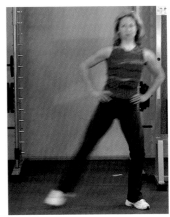

Plie Squat With Drag

What it does: Tones the inner and front thighs.

What you do: Stand with good posture, feet wider than hip width, toes and knees at 45°, hands on the thighs. Draw up through your abdominals. Bend the knees, lowering the torso towards the floor. Keep the weight on your heels and your spine in neutral position, tail bone pointing down as you lower. Draw your weight on to one leg as you drag the other leg towards it. Use your inner thighs to draw the legs together. Draw the legs apart and repeat on the other side.

How many? 12–16 on each leg

Back

Body Kit

Resitance band/tubing

Exercise ball or chair

Mat

Pilates bed

Lat pull-down machine

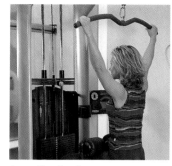 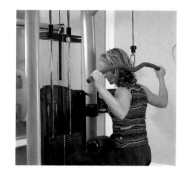

Lat Pull-down

What it does: Tones the large upper back muscle.

What you do: Sit facing the weight stack on the lat pull-down machine. Check the weight pin is on an appropriate weight for you. With a wide grip hold the bar. Ensure the shoulders are down before you pull the bar down. Draw in the elbows towards the waist as you lower the bar down towards the top of the neck. Keep the abdominals contracted as you lower. Slowly let the bar return to the start position, keeping the shoulders down.

Top Tip: Imagine keeping a distance between your ears and your shoulders. This will help you keep the shoulder girdle stabilized as you complete this exercise.

How many? 8–12

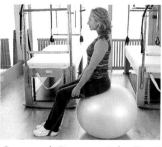 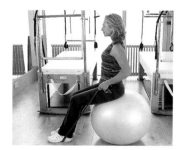

Seated Row with Resistance Band

What it does: Improves posture and tightens the upper trapezius muscles.

What you do: Sit with good posture on an exercise ball or chair. Place a resistance band under your feet and hold on to each end with arms slightly extended. Draw the elbows back towards you close by your side (imagine squeezing a lemon between your shoulder blades as you do this) and then return to the start position.

How many? 12–16

Top Tip: Different bands have different resistance, so choose one to suit you, and adjust your hand position to get the right tension.

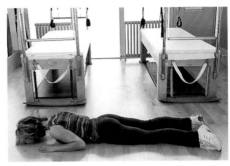 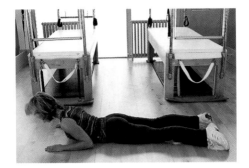

Cobra With Arm Support

What it does: Strengthens the long back extensor muscles.

What you do: Lie on the floor face down, hands by your shoulders. Slowly lift your head and upper body off the floor, supporting your weight with your hands. Keep the neck in line and lengthen through the crown of the head as you lift. Keep the abdominals contracted as you lift. Slowly lower down to the floor. As you get stronger, take less weight in your hands. This will help your back extensor muscles work harder.

How many? 8–10

Top Tip: Rotating the feet outwards when on the floor will help support your lower back.

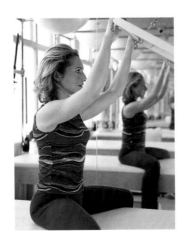 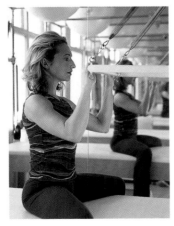

Inclined Trapezius Pull-ins

What it does: Strengthens the lower back and tones the upper trapezius muscles.

What you do: Sit on a Pilates bed, legs extended and back in neutral position. Extend back from the hips, keeping the spine in a neutral position and your abdominals firmly contracted to support your spine. Ensure your ribs are down. Draw a spring-loaded bar towards your chest, keeping the elbows wide. Return the bar to the start position and straighten your back.

How many? 6–8

Top Tip: This is a challenging exercise. Make sure your ribcage stays low (see page 77). If you do not have access to a Pilates bed, this exercise can also be done with a piece of tubing placed over the top of a door frame.

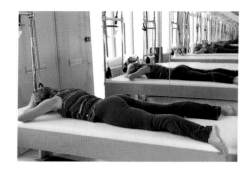 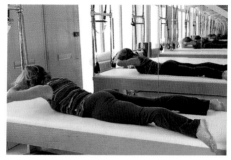 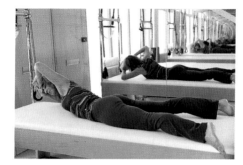

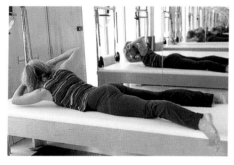 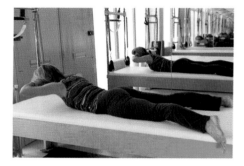

Back Extension With Rotation

What it does: Gives balance and tone to the spinal rotating muscles.

What you do: Lie face down, fingers resting on your forehead. Keep the abdominals contracted as you slowly lift the upper body off the floor. Keep the eye-line down. Slowly rotate the upper body, turning your shoulders to one side. Return to the central position and then lower. Repeat, rotating the body to the other side.

How many? 8–10

Top Tip: If you find this exercise too challenging, build up to it by keeping your hands on the floor as you rotate.

Strength training can reduce the risk of osteoporosis, and it can also play an important part in the management of it. (See page 88 for a specific osteoporosis case study.) You may be completely new to strength training – and also short of time! So, if you can't manage anything else, here are the 3 essential exercises you should do as a safeguard against diminishing bone density.

Body Kit
Resistance band
Hand weights
Bench

Workout
1 set of these 3 exercises per session is sufficient.

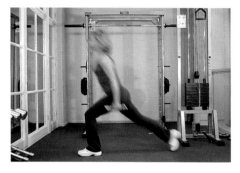

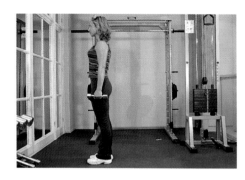

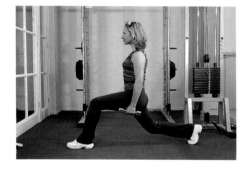

Lunge

Why: A compound strength exercise that challenges all the muscles of the lower leg and encourages bone-loading in the lower limbs. Add dumbbells in each hand to increase weight-bearing.

What it does: Tones the quadriceps, hamstrings, buttocks and calves.

What you do: Stand with good posture. Taking a large stride, extend one leg back. The front knee should be over the front ankle and the back leg should be long with a slight bend at the knee. Keep the back knee and heel off the floor. Contract through the abdominals as you lift yourself back up to a straight position. Change legs.

How many? Build up to 12

Top Tip: To help with your balance, contract up through the pelvic floor muscles as you lift.

Bench Press

Why: Strengthens the upper body and stabilizes the spine, as it increases the bone density of the upper body.

What it does: Targets the shoulders, biceps and chest.

What you do: Lie on your back with knees bent and feet either on the bench or the floor. Make sure you have neutral alignment through your spine. Hold the dumbbells with your elbows bent at shoulder level and press them up over the chest, then lower to the start position. Make sure the elbows do not drop lower than chest level.

How many? Build up to 12

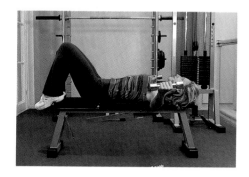 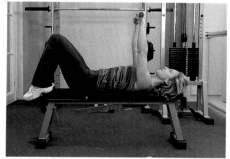

Frontal Raise

Why: Stimulates muscle contraction at shoulder and elbow joints and strengthens the arms (a particularly weak area for women). Strengthening the arms and increasing bone density in the upper limbs reduces the risk of serious injury from falls.

What it does: Shapes the front of the shoulder and tones the long head of the biceps muscle.

What you do: Stand with good posture. Palms up, hold a weighted body bar in front of you. Keeping the back straight and the abdominals contracted, lift the arms to eye-level. Keep a slight bend at the elbow. Slowly lower down.

Top Tip: No body bar? Create your own with a broom handle and two old nylon tights each filled with 2.25kg/5lb of pebbles. Making sure they are an equal distance apart, secure the filled tights with binding tape to either end of the broom handle.

How many? Build up to 12

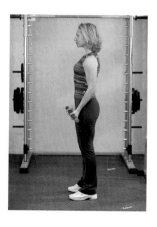 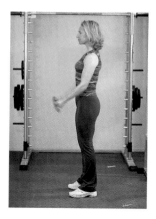 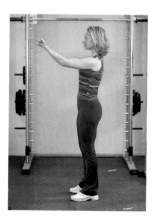

Questions and answers

Q As a woman, I've always been put off strength training as I believed it would make my muscles large and bulky. Is this true?

A Strength training will result in a small increase in the total muscle mass. However, large increases in muscle size will not result because testosterone levels, which are associated with muscle bulk, are lower in the female than in the male. Genetic factors and individual differences will mean that some women see a greater increase in their muscle mass than others – but nowhere near the muscle size of men.

Q Will I be able to increase my strength as much as my boyfriend?

A Studies have shown women can experience as much strength gain as men. Some studies have actually shown greater strength increases in women compared to men. However, these strength gains are relative, as women have less muscle mass than men to begin with.

Q I am older and not used to doing weight training – do I need to start now?

A Older women must participate in activities specifically designed to strengthen all muscle groups if they want to maintain maximum health and quality of lifestyle. There are many health benefits of strength training, including reduced risk of osteoporosis, decreased risk of injury and sustained physical independence later in life.

Q Do I have to join a gym to perform strength-training exercises?

A No. As long as your muscles are brought to a point of overload you can use a whole variety of equipment to improve your strength. An inexpensive strength training kit will include dumbbells, ankle weights, resistance bands, barbells and your own body weight (see equipment to use on page 66).

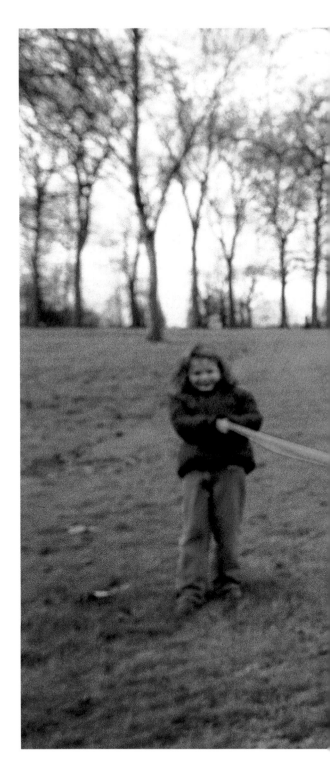

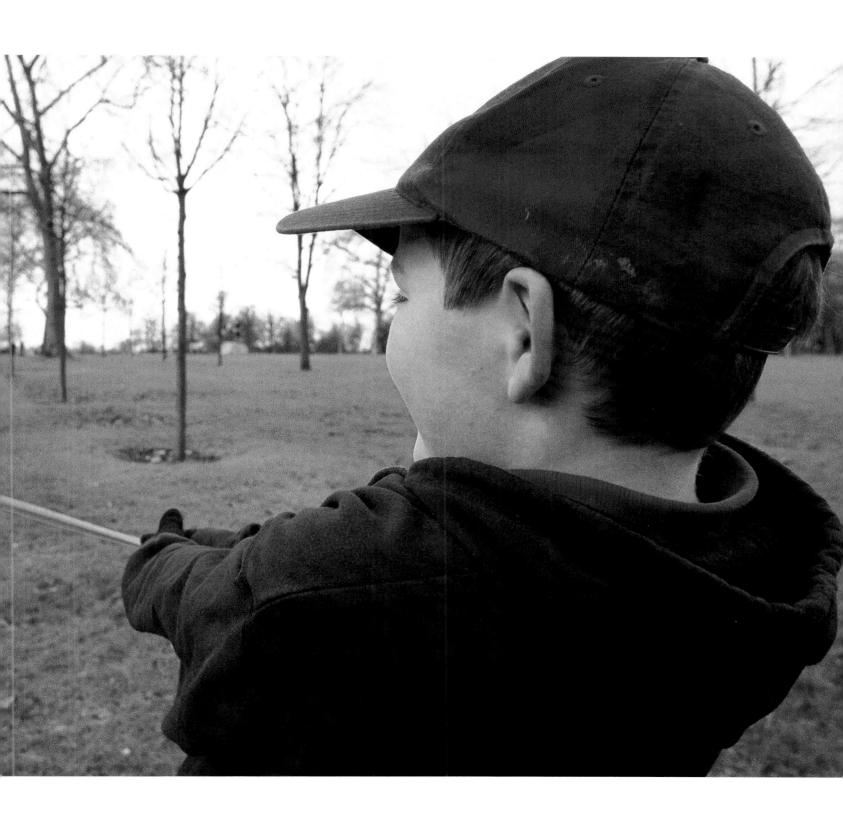

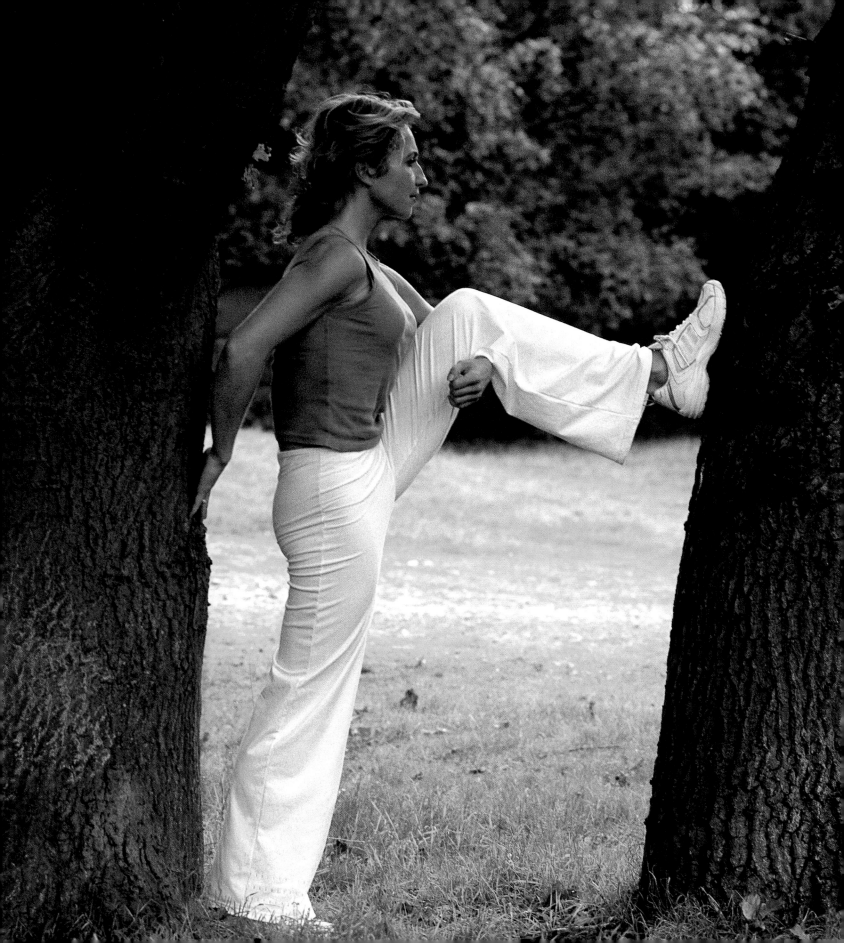

flexibility

Flexibility, balance and co-ordination should form a key part of your programme, helping you to achieve a fit, healthy and poised body. All too often, we skip the stretching routine through lack of time, or because we believe we have already reaped the benefits of our training with the sweat and toil of the cardiovascular and resistance part of our workouts. However, the increasing popularity of mind-body exercises such as yoga, t'ai chi and Pilates is now highlighting the fundamental role mobility, stretching and balance should play in our total body wellbeing.

A flexibility programme should aim to optimize mobility and enhance elasticity of your muscles, whilst maintaining the stability of the joints. So next time you feel like skipping out of your exercise class early, here are some reasons to make sure you don't miss out on those all-important stretches – to save time you can even do them in the changing rooms as you are getting dressed!

Why you should stretch

Age

Like it or not, as we age our flexibility tends to decrease because we lose elasticity in the connective tissue surrounding the muscles. Couple this with an inactive lifestyle and you will find yourself with limited mobility.

Exercise

When we move, the muscles naturally shorten and contract. Even continual movement in everyday life, without flexibility work, can lead to residual shortening of muscle tissue and connective ligaments, leaving our bodies feeling stiffer, causing muscular imbalances and reducing our range of movement.

Joints

You may be flexible in one part of your body, but this is not indicative of your overall flexibility levels. Flexibility is specific to each joint and its particular structure. So it is important to adopt a 'whole body' approach to your flexibility and mobility. Even if you are able to wrap your left leg around the back of your head, you may still need to address the mobility of your spine or ankle joints.

Pregnancy

During pregnancy the pelvic joints and ligaments are relaxed and capable of a greater range of motion. This is due to the increased secretion of the hormone relaxin. Its effects can be felt up to 6 months after the baby is born, at which point relaxin production tends to decease and the ligaments tighten up. again. (See page 145 for more information on how your body changes during pregnancy.)

The benefits of stretching

A flexibility and mobility programme:

1. **Increases the functional range of motion of each joint.**

   A limited range of motion in certain joints may not particularly bother you when your muscles are young and flexible, but think about when you are older, and may not be able to reach to the top shelf in the kitchen cupboard, or bend comfortably to tie up your shoes. Or maybe you have difficulty unzipping your dress at the back and you have to ask someone to help you. Such problems stem from a limited range of motion.

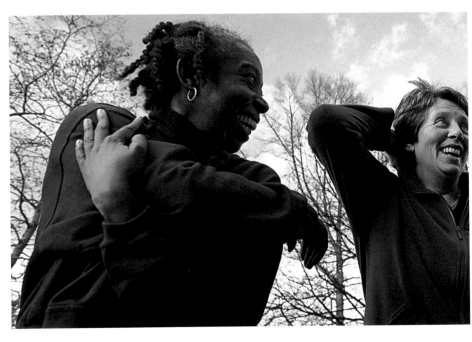

2. **Reduces low back pain and risk of injury.**
Back pain is one of the most common disabilities affecting our society today. It accounts for a loss of 5 million working days a year. And it is attributed to muscular imbalance in the trunk muscles and inappropriate flexibility in the pelvis. (See the Mobility Programme on page 99).

3. **Decreases the severity of a potential injury.**
Watch any downhill alpine skier take one of those spectacular falls and you will soon see that optimal flexibility can reduce the seriousness of injuries. You may not be an Olympic skier, but having good flexibility can minimize the damage you can experience even from a simple fall.

4. **Improves your body's posture and symmetry.**
Muscular imbalances, through shortening and differential strength in the torso, create misalignment of the skeletal system and the consequent development of rounded shoulders, poor posture and dowager's hump (a condition in which the upper back becomes severely rounded). (For tips on how to improve your posture, see Better Posture Workout, page 102)

5. **Delays the onset of muscle fatigue.**
Taking the muscles through their range of motion before an intense workout allows you to do more before you start to feel tired, making the workouts more enjoyable and effective.

6. **Reduces or prevents muscle soreness after exercise.**
The soreness you experience in your muscles 24–48 hours post-workout may result from by micro-tears in the muscle fibres caused by over-exertion. While stretching does not directly repair micro-tears, it does help to maintain muscle elasticity, thereby reducing the risk of future damage. In addition, micro-tears lay down collagen as they heal, which is less elastic than muscle tissue. So stretch after your workouts – you will find all the essential muscle stretches on page 129–135). Regular stretching ensures a good range of motion throughout your whole body. If you have limited mobility it is a good idea to complete preparatory stretches that take the body through its full range of motion as part of your warm-up.

7. **Enhances feelings of calm and well-being.**
Practices such as yoga and t'ai chi focus on the inner breath and the link between the busy mind and stressed physical body. To help you feel calmer and less stressed, see the Relaxation Meditation on page 98.

8. **Provides an opportunity for stillness and spiritual growth.**
Devotees of mind-body fitness often report that they feel a greater sense of connection with their inner self.

Body laid bare

And now for the science bit...

When a muscle stretches, tiny receptors known as muscle spindles are stimulated and send a message to the spinal cord that the muscle is being extended. If the muscle is being extended too quickly and vigorously, the spinal cord sends a reflex message to the muscle to contract. This is the stretch reflex, one of your body's basic protective mechanisms to stop it over-stretching. This explains why bouncing in a stretch position, or ballistic stretching (see p. 96), can be detrimental and potentially damaging to the muscle tissue.

Located near the tendon muscle junction, the golgi tendon organ (GTO) is another sensory receptor. When excessive tension is created in the muscle from either a deep stretch or a muscle contraction, the GTO triggers a reflex known as the inverse stretch reflex. This reflex inhibits muscle contraction and relaxes the muscle. The GTO is therefore part of the body's very clever defence mechanism which prevents the muscle from developing too much tension, which may lead to injury.

Posture assessment

Good posture should be the foundation of all your movements, stress, long periods spent on the phone, sitting for hours at a time… all effect your posture.

To stand with good posture, place your weight evenly on both feet. Extend up through the thighs and feel the pelvis rest lightly on the tops of the thighs. Stretch up through the spine. Let the shoulders drop down and away from your ears. Soften the rib cage, drawing the bottom rib down towards your hips. It may help to imagine you are wearing a corset. Now contract the abdominals, drawing the navel in towards the back of the spine. You should feel balanced and relaxed in this position.

To check you are standing with good posture, here are some posture reference points:

Your pelvis position

Place the heel of the hand on the top of the hip bone (the iliac crest), and extend your fingertips down to the pubic bone. If you are standing with good posture, the fingertips and the heel of the hand should be directly on top of each other (see Neutral spine, below). Your fingertips should be neither in front of the heel of your hand (kyphotic alignment) nor behind it (lordotic alignment). Adjust your pelvis to realign your hand and hip position.
(To check your posture while you're sitting, see page 174 for the Seated Symmetry Test).

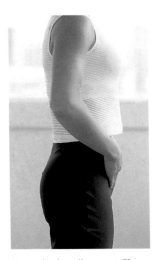 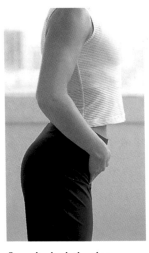 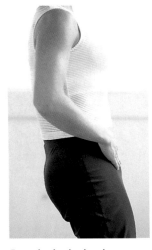

Neutral spine alignment. The pelvis is evenly stacked, sitting on top of each thigh bone.

Excessive lordotic spine alignment. This is characterised by the top of the iliac crest tilting forward as the tail bones roll backwards.

Excessive kyphotic spine alignment. Here, a flat back is created as the tail bones tilt forward.

Types of stretching

Stretching techniques are continually evolving, and at present there are no universally agreed guidelines to follow. However, for your flexibility to increase, you definitely need a slow and progressively increasing stretch, taking the muscle just past the point of limitation, but not to the point of pain.

There are various types of stretching techniques. Each is appropriate for different activities.

Ballistic

This type of stretching involves bouncing in the stretch position. Mainly used by athletes to simulate movements in sport, it is a stretching technique that can cause injury, and is generally considered less effective than other methods.

Static

The most commonly used flexibility technique, as it is very safe and effective, and most suitable for the recreational exerciser. With this technique, the muscle or muscle group is held in the position for up to 30 seconds.

Passive

This type of stretching is commonly practised with the aid of an object such as a towel, wall or bench. They can be very useful for someone with a limited range of flexibility.

Proprioceptive neuromuscular facilitation (PNF)

This is an advanced stretching technique, which has proved to be a very effective way of increasing your range of motion. Two commonly used techniques in PNF are:

Contract-relax:

1. Tense the targeted muscle so that you feel mild discomfort as it is taken to the point of feeling a stretch.
2. Start to contract statically the targeted muscle in the pre-stretched position for 4–6 seconds.
3. Relax the contracted muscle group and then stretch the muscle to a new point of limitation.

Contract-relax against contract:

This stretching technique is the most effective way to improve flexibility. Follow steps 1–3 as above. Then:

4. Contract the opposing muscles for 4–6 seconds against a resistance.
5. Now relax the primary muscle and take the targeted muscle to a point of further stretch.

Active isolated stretching

Studies have shown that the greater the difference between a contracting muscle and the range of motion of the opposing muscle group, the greater the likelihood of injury.

To find out which muscles are opposing each other, move your body. For example, bend your arm at the elbow to draw the hand up to your shoulder. The biceps is responsible for the movement, and to extend the arm back to the straight position the triceps muscle at the back of the arm has to contract.

You can follow this example of an active isolated stretch for the hamstrings.

1. Isolate the muscle group (the hamstrings, for example at the back of the thigh) to be stretched. Lie on the floor and draw the hamstrings into the chest with the leg straight.
2. Contract the opposing muscle group (the quadriceps – the muscle at the front of the thigh). To do this, focus on pulling the leg in towards the head using the quadriceps muscle.
3. Hold the quadriceps in a contracted position for 1–4 seconds and then relax. Feel the hamstrings as you do this.
4. Complete 8–12 repetitions.
5. Exhale on the stretch of each repetition.

Stretching Dos and Donts
So you've resolved not to skimp on your stretches? Here are a few pointers…

- **DO warm up before stretching.**
  The warm-up will increase the temperature of the ligaments, blood, tendons and muscles, allowing them to become more mobile and elastic.
- **DO perform stretches every day.**
  Stretching on a daily basis will improve your flexibility.
- **DO concentrate on the muscle you are stretching.**
  Focus on feeling a mild discomfort in the middle part of the muscle being stretched.

- **DO stretch the muscle in different positions.**
  The muscle tendons are attached to the bone at various sites. Stretching the muscle in different positions will provide a more effective stretch response and improve your overall range of motion, as well as preventing muscle boredom.
- **DO stretch after each strenuous workout.**
  It will relieve delayed onset of muscle soreness and aid relaxation.
- **DO NOT rush your stretches.**
  Move into the stretch positions slowly and always try to relax the targeted muscle before you stretch

- **DO NOT stretch beyond the point of pain.**
  While you should feel a stretch in the muscles you should not be in pain when it is under tension. If you feel pain, ease off the position, take a deep breath and ease into the position again to about 80% of the point of the previous stretch.
- **DO NOT hold your breath.**
  Breathing freely through the stretch position will enhance blood flow to the muscle area and reduce the risk of elevated blood pressure.

Relaxation Meditation

Many people find stretching can be very relaxing. Combining it with a deep relaxing meditation can be a great way to ease your mind and enhance the depth of stretch you can achieve with your body. Try this meditation in conjunction with your stretching programme.

This meditation will aid restful sleep and help quiet a tense body and busy brain.

You may wish to recite this passage and record it on a CD or audiotape to play it when you want to relax and unwind. Alternatively you can work with a friend to help you relax.

Lie on the floor, palms up and arms slightly away from the body. Inhale deeply, and on exhalation allow your body to sink into the floor. Close your eyes for peace and quiet. Focus on the even flow of your breath.

Relax your body from head to toe. Every time you hear the word RELAX, try to relax your brain, body and mind completely. Be still. RELAX – RELAX – RELAX.

RELAX your body. Concentrate on relaxing the top of the head. Feel a wave of stillness, calmness and relaxation wash over your body. Start with your forehead; then the tiny muscles around your eyes. Think about your cheeks and then your mouth. Smile softly inside to yourself. Move your jaw a little to release any tension that might be there. Now draw attention down to your neck and your shoulders. Turn your head slowly to one side and then the other. Press your shoulder blades into the back of the floor and release. Let go of any tension in this area.

RELAX and let go. RELAX. Feel a wave of stillness, calmness and relaxation wash down over your arms and hands. Slowly wriggle your fingers, feel softness in your fingertips. Breathe in and exhale deeply. Listen to your breath. RELAX the rib cage, allow the ribs to fall further into the floor with each breath. RELAX.

Feel a wave of stillness, calmness and relaxation wash down through your abdomen and internal organs. Visualize your breath moving in and out of your body. RELAX.

Feel a wave of stillness, calmness and relaxation wash down through your pelvic area. Let the hips sink into the floor. You now feel at peace and still. RELAX. Feel a wave of stillness, calmness and relaxation wash down through your legs, down your calves and feet. Feel the calmness flood into your toes. RELAX. RELAX and let go. RELAX. You are now feeling calm, peaceful and still.

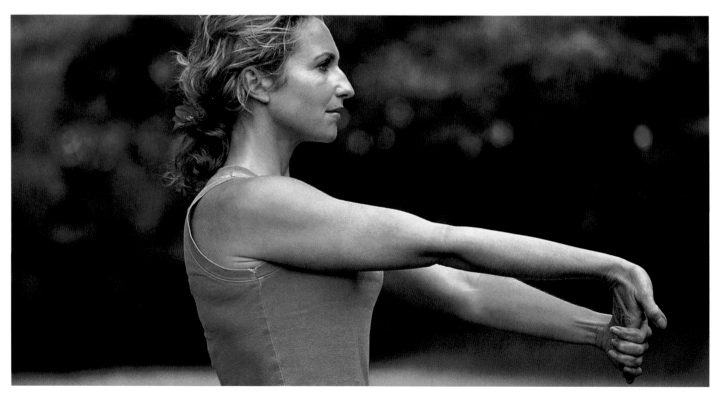

This is a simple workout that will take you less than 10 minutes. Try it first thing in the morning to relieve stiffness after sleep. While you are asleep the limited mobility of the body can cause the joints to stiffen as the joint fluid is cooler. This workout will help waken your body and warm the elasticity of your joints.

When stretching, your body may cool down, so it is often a good idea to add a layer to maintain your body temperature.

Body Kit

Chair, bed or bench

Mat or rug

Warm clothing

The Workout

Seated Spine Rotation x 4 right and left

Full Body Stretch x 2

Lying Spine Stretch x 2 right and left

Cat Curl x 4

Opposite Arm and Leg Reach x 4 right and left

Side Bend x 8 right and left

Wall Roll-down x 6

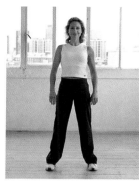 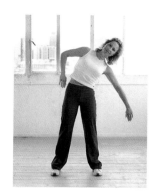

Side Bend

What it does: Mobilizes the lower spine.

What you do: Stand with your feet hip-distance apart, with your weight evenly distributed between both feet. Bend your knees slightly to reduce the pressure on your spine. With your abdominals contracted and your spine long, gently slide your hand down the side of your leg to feel a stretch on your waist. To avoid leaning forwards, imagine you are going down between two panes of glass, one in front of you and one behind. Keep your shoulders back and over your hips. Keep the lower body still.

How many? Repeat in a controlled manner, up to 8 times each side.

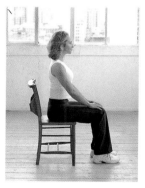 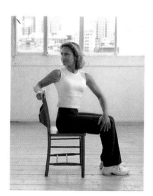

Seated Spine Rotation

What it does: Releases tension in the middle back.

What you do: Sit up tall on a chair or on the side of your bed. Your feet need to be flat on the floor and directly under your knees. Place your right hand on the outside of your left thigh and reach back with your left hand. Be tall as you turn. You can use your hands as levers to increase the stretch you feel.

How long? Stretch only to a comfortable position, holding for 10–15 seconds. Repeat 4 times on each side.

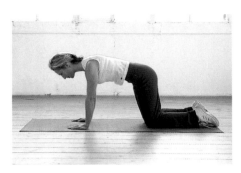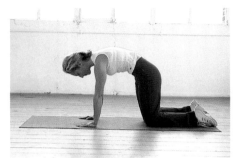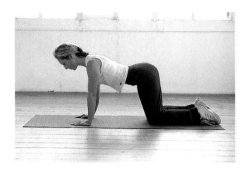

Cat Curl

What it does: An excellent stretch for mobilizing the spine.

What you do: Start on all fours, with your wrists under your shoulders and your knees directly under your hips. Contract your abdominals to arch the back up to the ceiling like a witch's cat. Pay particular attention to the lumbar region of the back and try to get as much stretch through this area as possible. Contract the abdominals and come back to a flat-back position. Imagine you could put a tray of drinks on your back. Next, in a controlled manner, let the lumbar spine arch to the floor and your tail bone point to the ceiling.

How many? Repeat 4–8 times in a controlled manner

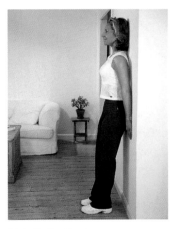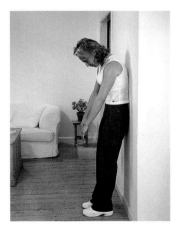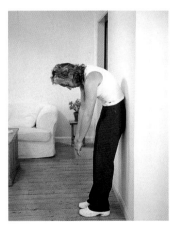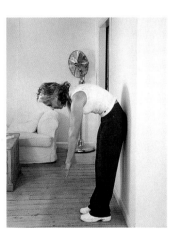

Wall Roll-down

What it does: Mobilizes the spine.

What you do: Stand with your back to a wall so that the whole length of your spine touches it. Ensure your lumbar vertebrae are in contact with the wall. You may find you need to have your feet about 30cm/12in away from the wall to achieve this. Slowly peel down the wall one vertebra at a time until you feel a stretch on the backs of your legs. Draw in through the abdominals to peel your back up the wall again, one vertebra at a time. This appears a simple exercise but discipline is required to ensure you peel just one vertebra at a time.

How many? 6

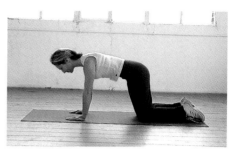 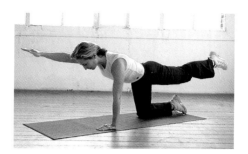

Opposite Arm and Leg Reach

What it does: Strengthens and tones the back and abdominal muscles.

What you do: Get on to all fours with your knees under your hips and your wrists directly under your shoulders. Have your back as flat as possible and strongly contract the abdominals to support the spine and create good balance. Slowly reach forwards with one arm and at the same time reach back with the opposite leg. Pulling in your abdominal muscles will help you keep your balance. Slowly bring your leg and arm back to the floor and repeat on the other side.

How many? Repeat 4–8 times on each side.

Top Tip: If you are new to this exercise, or feel unsteady supporting your weight on one hand and one leg, perform the same leg and arm reaches lying on the floor. Make sure you keep looking down to the floor as you reach. As you get stronger, move on to the all-fours position.

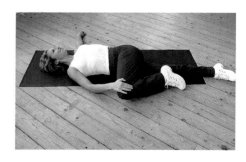

Lying Spine Stretch

What it does: Releases tension in the lower spine, which is especially important if you sit at a desk or spend a lot of time in a car.

What you do: Lie on the floor face-up with your legs extended. Lift one knee towards the chest and gently ease it across the opposite side of your body, supporting with the opposite hand. As far as possible keep the knee at 90° to the torso. You are aiming to get the inside of the knee to the floor on the other side of your body. Breathe in a controlled manner and do only what is comfortable for you. To change sides contract the abdominals and release the leg to the floor.

How long? Hold for up to 30 seconds on each side and and repeat.

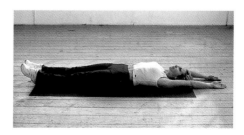

Full Body Stretch

What it does: Stretches the whole of the body, especially the abdominal and spine area.

What you do: Lie on the floor face-up. Extend your arms above your head. Gently stretch and lengthen through your whole body from your fingertips to your toes. Your lower back may come gently off the floor. Slowly bring your arms down by your side. Breathe gently.

How long? Hold the extended position for up to 30 seconds and repeat.

Our posture says a lot about us. It conveys our levels of self-esteem and our ability to move with minimum risk of injury. Our daily life challenges our body to cope with many things such as stress, long periods of being in one position and carrying bags that place more load on one side than the other. This workout is designed to get you back in tune with your posture, correct general muscle imbalances, stabilize your spine and increase the strength of the core trunk muscles.

Body Kit

Resistance band

Wall

Belt

The Workout

Assess your posture first (see page 96).

Wall Roll-down x 6

Resistance Band Shoulder Pull x 6

Belt Tuck x 8

Hip Flexor Stretch x 1 right and left

Prone Shoulder Opening x 12

Back Raise With Arm Extension x 8

Wall Roll-down x 8

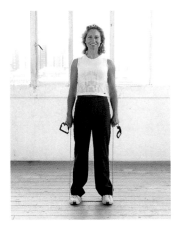 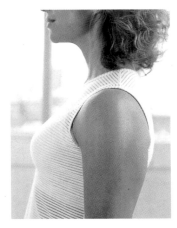

Resistance Band Shoulder Pull

What it does: A very subtle yet effective exercise that lengthens the neck and draws the shoulders down away from ears.

What you do: Stand with both feet on a reisistance band. Hold the resistance band so you feel the tension of the band gently pulling your shoulders down. This is your start position. Now try to use your back muscles to lower the shoulders further. Aim to minimize the pull of the band and loosen the tension. Hold for 10 seconds and relax.

How many? 6

Top Tip: As you get more confident with this exercise, challenge yourself to contract your pelvic floor muscles while you are contracting through your back muscles.

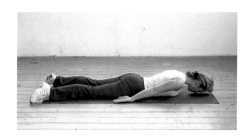 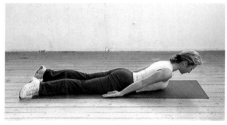 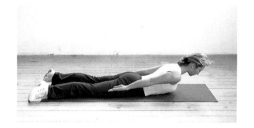

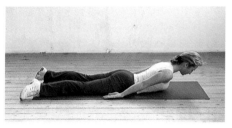 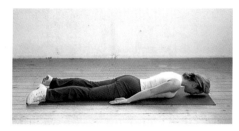

Back Raise With Arm Extension

What it does: Strengthens the trunk muscles and opens the shoulder girdle.

What you do: There are 4 parts to this exercise. Lie face-down, forehead resting on the floor and arms down by your sides. Lift your upper body off the floor, stretching your fingertips to your toes. Raise your arms towards the ceiling and then lower them down to the floor and lower your upper body.

How many? 8–12

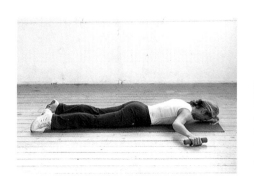 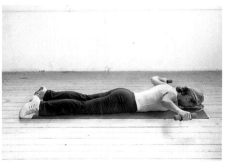

Prone Shoulder Opening

What it does: Opens the shoulder area, particularly beneficial if breast-feeding or spending a lot of time in front of the computer.

What you do: Lie face-down, arms spread out to the side level with the shoulders. Keep the palms facing down and head in contact with the floor. Lift the arms from the shoulders off the floor, imagining you are squeezing a lemon between your shoulder blades, then lower the arms.

How many? 8–12

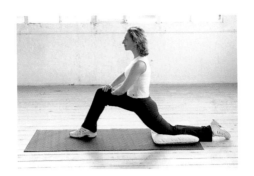

Hip Flexor Stretch

What it does: The hip flexors are among the strongest muscles in the body; when they get short, they tend to pull on the lumbar spine and can compress the vertebra discs, causing pain. The hip flexor stretch helps prevent this.

What you do: Come into a lunge position. Make sure your front knee is over your ankle and your knee cap is in line with your second toe. Extend the back leg, pressing the pelvis down to the floor. You may need to use your hands for support.

How long? Hold for 10–30 seconds. Repeat on the other side

Belt Tuck

What it does: When the abdominals weaken, they lack the ability to provide support for the spine, and this can cause lordosis of the spine (see page 96). This exercise is a very simple way to prevent this and to start to develop some muscle tone. It is particularly beneficial as it supports the body in the way we most commonly need it to work – in an upright position!

What you do: Stand wearing a belt fastened firmly around the waist. Maintaining good posture, try to slide your fingertips in between the belt and your skin. To do this, draw the abdominal wall into the back of your spine, pulling in the tummy button as you contract. Hold for 15 seconds while breathing smoothly and make sure you keep the rib cage relaxed as you contract your abdominals.

How many? 8–20

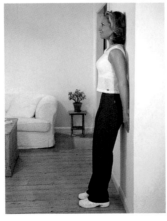
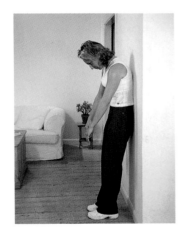
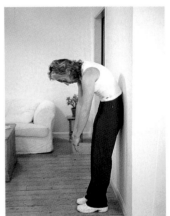
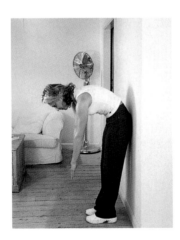

Wall Roll-down

What it does: This is a great exercise for easing stiffness in the spine.

What you do: Stand with your back to a wall so that the length of your spine is in contact with it. Ensure your lumbar vertebrae are in contact with the wall. You may find you need to have your feet about 30cm/12in away from the wall to achieve this. Slowly peel down the wall one vertebra at a time until you feel a stretch on the backs of your legs. Draw in through the abdominals to peel your back up the wall again, one vertebra at a time. This appears a simple exercise but it takes discipline to ensure that you peel one vertebra at a time.

How many: 4–8

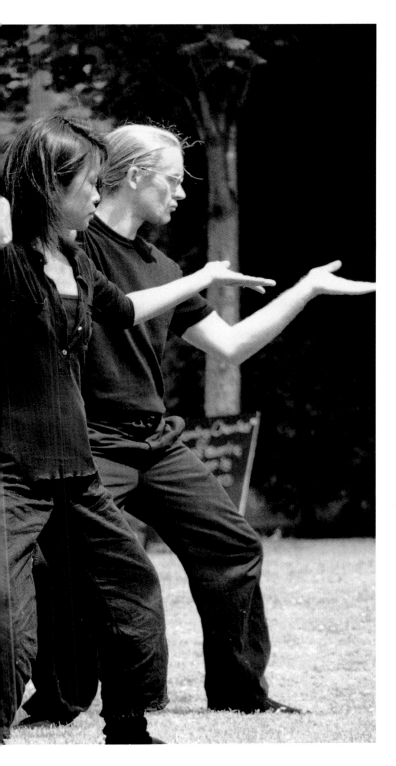

Techniques and workouts: flexibility, balance and co-ordination

Pressures of modern living have made Eastern mind-body practices very popular with Westerners. More health clubs and local communities are providing t'ai chi and yoga classes than ever before. You will find a variety of workouts here, drawing upon different disciplines such as t'ai chi and Pilates. If you have not tried this type of exercise before – try it – all will enhance your body's mobility and flexibility. and give peace of mind.

T'ai chi ch'uan

T'ai chi ch'uan is the ancient Chinese art of moving meditation. It is based on the Taoist understanding that all things are made up of two complementary forces – Yin and Yang.

With its distinctive grace and flowing movements, t'ai chi ch'uan is becoming an increasingly popular form of relaxation in the West, providing an effective antidote to our stressful and often competitive society. Many people practise t'ai chi solely for its benefit to health and as a means to relieve tension. However, t'ai chi is a complete training, and is often referred to as meditation in movement. Devotees believe the calmness and stillness experienced in t'ai chi is greater than the stillness attained in stillness itself.

T'ai chi ch'uan is also an effective martial art – its name translates as 'supreme ultimate boxing'. To attain this level of understanding, however, takes many years of dedicated study and practice, and consequently it is not suitable for a person whose sole concern is self-defence. If this is your primary interest, try Tai Kwon Do, karate or judo

Consistent and diligent practice of t'ai chi will restore your mind and spirit to their original state of integrity. T'ai chi reconnects the mind to the body, the conscious to the unconscious and the individual to their environment.

There are many different styles of t'ai chi ch'uan, but the most widespread are the Chen, the Yang and the Wu. There are variations within these styles, and there are also different styles of teaching within these variations. If the first classes that you attend are not to your taste, don't lose heart, but keep looking. The first four exercises outlined here are not style-specific, and can help you along until you find a good teacher.

Basic principles

Breathing

For the first few years of t'ai chi the focus is on mastering the natural breath. To do this, begin by letting go of tension in the chest and shoulders, then use the mind to soften the front of the body. Gradually the solar plexus and belly relax, the diaphragm is allowed to drop and the breath begins to come from the lower abdomen instead of from the chest. Breathing comes naturally, without deliberate muscular effort, from the *tan tien* – an area 5–7.5cm/2–3in below the navel and one third of the way in from the front of the body. Focusing the awareness here automatically regulates the breath in the correct way. Followers of t'ai chi believe The *tan tien* is a centre for subtle energy, and a focus for meditation. It is also the centre of gravity of the physical body.

Relaxation

In t'ai chi, the art of relaxation is achieved by what is called a softening and opening of the mind. All of the tension and strength in the upper body is allowed to sink down to the soles of the feet and then into the ground. This results in the settling of the *chi* (the invisible energy force that flows throught the body), and a firm grounding of one foot at all times.

The waist

All movements in t'ai chi are centred in the *tan tien* and hips, and this area is referred to as the waist. The t'ai chi waist can be likened to a wheel rotating around a central axle, represented in the spine. The 'oil' that enables this 'wheel' to turn freely is supplied by the mind. There is a connection between the hips and shoulders on each side – when the hips turn, the shoulders turn at the same time and by the same amount, no more, no less. At beginner and intermediate levels, there is no twisting of the spine – it is as if the torso is a cylinder standing on its end rotating around a central axis.

The exercises

The first four of the following exercises can be practised each day as a set. Initially spend 8–10 minutes doing the exercises, then gradually extend the time – little and often is much better than a lot once in a while. Finish your practice by sitting comfortably on an upright chair, with your feet parallel, your hands gently clasped and resting in your lap. Spend 1–2 minutes listening to your natural breath. The opening postures of the Yang style form can be attempted when you are feeling more comfortable with the first exercises.

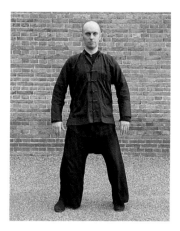 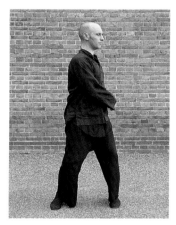 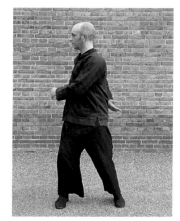

Knocking at the Gates of Heaven

What it does: This will stimulate your natural energy (*chi*), calm your mind, and help release excess tension in your body. Sinking your awareness down to your *tan tien* helps to quieten a busy mind, and also regulates the natural breath. Sitting and sinking into the legs improves your connection to the ground, and with practice you will notice that your balance is gradually improving.

What you do: Stand with your feet parallel, shoulder-width apart. Imagine that the soles of your feet are melting into the ground. The knees are bent and gently pushed away from each other so that the insteps of your feet feel as if

they are made from cotton wool. Gently tuck in your bottom so that you are sitting in your legs rather than standing on them, so there is a sense that the sacrum is connected to the ground. Do not clench your buttocks.

The chest and shoulders are completely relaxed, as are the arms which hang naturally by the sides. The chin is tucked in, gently, the lips and teeth are lightly held together and the tip of the tongue is held against the top palate slightly behind the teeth. Do not lean or incline your upper body in any direction, but stand with a vertical and natural posture as if suspended from a thread attached to the crown of your head.

Turn your waist to the left, sit in your left leg and sink 70% of your weight down into the sole of your left foot. Turn your waist to the right, sit in your right leg and sink 70% of your weight down into the sole of your right foot. In a continuous movement, the waist turns smoothly to the left and to the right while the hips remain level throughout. Turn the waist as far as you can without forcing the limits of your flexibility, and keep softening your hips and keep your bottom tucked in. As the waist turns, the weight moves from one leg to the other as if the legs were hollow and the weight is a liquid that fills them up.

This rotation of your torso mobilizes your arms which, as they are relaxed, turn freely with the rest of your body. At the end of each waist turn, as the waist is changing direction, the arms strike the front and back of your body at the height of the *tan tien*. Throughout the exercise, keep your arms completely relaxed, like ropes, and try to avoid making any deliberate movements with them.

As you begin to settle into a relaxed and unhurried tempo, sink your awareness down to your *tan tien* and the soles of your feet, and observe the natural breath.

How long? Continue for 5 minutes

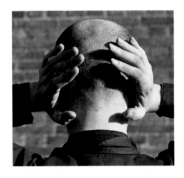
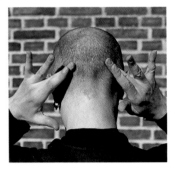
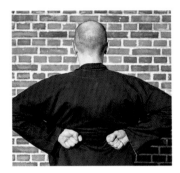
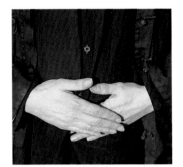

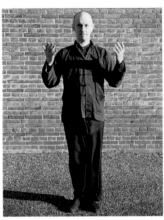
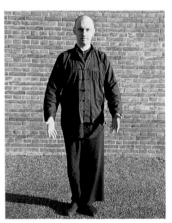

Massage Points and Chi Kung

What it does: This stimulates some important energy centres in the body, and is followed by some gentle chi kung (an exercise that promotes the free and natural flow of *chi*).

What you do: Stand as before, except this time the heels are touching and the toes are turned out so that the feet are at 45˚. The legs are straight but the knees are not locked. With the palms press firmly, but not forcefully, on the ears, then pull the palms away.

How many? Repeat 24 times.

What you do: Flick the forefingers off the middle fingers, quite firmly, on to 2 points which are found at the base of the skull, just to the outside of the 2 tendons located there.

How many? Repeat 24 times.

What you do: Form 2 soft fists and massage the kidney area of the back, quite firmly, using a circular motion – with the mind, visualize that you are drawing energy up from the sacrum to the kidneys. Keep your shoulders relaxed.

How many? Repeat for 36 circles.

What you do: Using the palms, rub the area of the *tan tien* and pelvis with circular motions. Completely relax the belly and keep the hands soft.

How many? Do 24 circles in one direction and then 24 in the other.

What you do: Be aware of the sensation in your palms. The lips and teeth are gently held together, and the tip of the tongue is held lightly against the top palate. Breathe through the nose. On the in-breath the mind 'pulls' on the sensation in the palms and the palms rise, arms bending at the elbows. On the out-breath allow the palms to 'fall'. This should feel as if the mind and the breath are moving the arms, so keep the arms and hands as relaxed as possible and use the bare minimum of muscular effort. The breath is relaxed, long and smooth.

How many? Repeat for 12 breaths

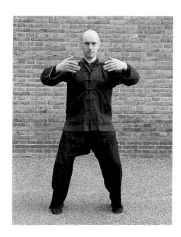

Holding the Urn

What it does: At first, do not spend too long on this exercise and over-strain yourself, but gradually increase the time you spend holding the posture. The benefits are similar to those of the first exercise. With time, you will begin to feel more stable and as your connection to the ground improves you will begin to form a 'root'. As your 'root' develops you will begin to feel more 'grounded' on many levels – physically, energetically and psychologically.

What you do: As before, stand with feet parallel, shoulder-width apart, knees bent and gently pushed away from each other. Without clenching your buttocks or the muscles in your lower abdomen, breathe out and tuck in your bottom until your sacrum is hanging vertically. Many t'ai chi students find this quite difficult at first, but with practice it gets easier. Do the best that you can without using too much muscular force – the secret is to soften and relax the structures around the hip joints gradually. The posture of the lower body is very similar to that when sitting on a horse.

Breathe out and imagine the soles of your feet melting into the ground. Check that your weight is evenly distributed between the front and back of each foot. If the insteps of your feet are collapsing into the ground, gently move the knees away from each other.

Hold the hands at chest height, with the palms shoulder-width apart and facing the body. Make the arms as round as possible from the centre of the back to the tips of the fingers, and imagine that you are holding a giant urn. Use just enough muscular effort to hold the shape in the arms. Allow the elbows to hang down slightly, as if there were weights hanging from them. Feel lightness in the hands, and keep the chest and shoulders as relaxed as possible.

Sink two thirds of your weight into your left leg and hold this posture for as long as you can, then sink your weight two thirds into your right leg. Again hold for as long as you can. Stop, relax your body, shake your arms and legs, then repeat.

Whilst holding the posture, try to let go of tension in the body. Sink your awareness down into the *tan tien* and the soles of your feet. Imagine that your legs have sunk into the ground up to your knees. Practise natural breathing.

How long? With a little regular practice you will soon be able to hold this posture for a few minutes in each leg. As you keep letting go of tension you may notice some unusual, but pleasant, sensations arising in your body – apart from your protesting thigh muscles!

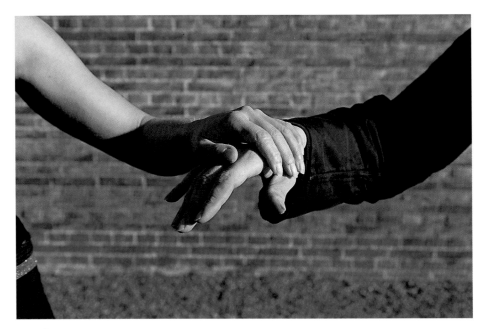

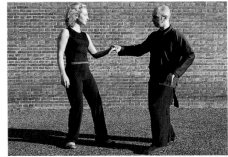

Sticking

What it does: Partnerwork is a very important part of t'ai chi, for it is here that we begin to learn about energy from other sources and our relationship to these energies. Through the practice of 'sticking' we can gain insights into the art of listening.

What you do: For this exercise you will need the help of a friend. First, decide who is going to lead (Person A) and who is going to follow (Person B). Person A holds up their right arm, palm facing the ground, and the person following places their left palm on top of the leader's hand.

Person A keeps their eyes open and person B has their eyes closed.

Person A then moves, in a relaxed manner, to wherever they like. The task for person B is to keep their palm lightly connected to person A and to follow their movements wherever they go.

When following, try to resist the urge to predict your partner's movements – listen, through your sense of touch, and remain lightly connected to what is actually happening. If your partner gets too close for comfort take a relaxed and natural step back. If they get too far away, instead of leaning or over-extending your arm, step forward.

Both people should keep their knees slightly bent, their posture relaxed and their movements natural.

How long? After a couple of minutes, change hands – B's right hand now following A's left. After another couple of minutes reverse roles.

The secret of sticking is to calm your mind, forget yourself, relax and listen.

Opening Postures of the Yang Style

Learning a t'ai chi form solely from words and pictures is a very difficult thing to do – instruction from a qualified teacher is the best approach. Until you find a class that suits you, have a go at these opening movements of the Yang style form. The instructions here have been simplified. Learning a complete form usually takes about a year of regular classes; the form is the foundation for the practice of moving meditation.

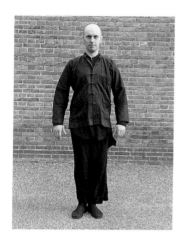

Posture 1: Attention

As before, stand with your heels touching and your toes turned out at 45°. Your legs are straight but your knees are not locked. Gently tuck your bottom in and relax your shoulders, chest and abdomen. Keep the tip of your tongue lightly held against the top palate, slightly behind your teeth, and breathe naturally through your nose down into the *tan tien*. Gently tuck in your chin and imagine that you are hanging from a thread attached to the crown of your head.

Allow the mind to soften, and all thoughts and tensions to flow down from your head to the soles of your feet. The sinking of the mind is accompanied by relaxation, an opening of the mind and a softening and a quietening of the body.

Posture 2: Preparation

Sink your weight down into the sole of your right foot, lift your left foot off the ground and place it, toes facing the front, shoulder-width from the right. Shift 70% of your weight into your left leg and square your hips to the front, pulling your right toes around so that they also face the front.

As you do this, your hands circle out from your body and then return to it, palms facing the ground and sitting on 'cushions of air', elbows slightly bent and shoulders relaxed.

Your legs are straight but your knees are not locked.

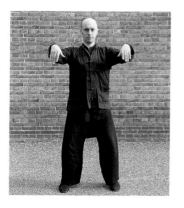

Posture 3: Beginning

Keep your weight 70% in your left leg. Relax your wrists completely as you raise both arms to shoulder-height, shoulder-width apart. Your arms are straight but your elbows are not locked.

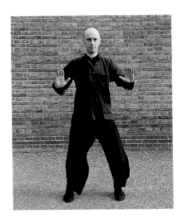

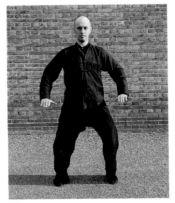

Bend your elbows and draw your hands towards your body, fingers pointing to the front as if they are floating off in water. Begin to lower your arms, and as you do so, bend your wrists slightly so that your palms face the front. Continue to lower your arms, your palms naturally turning to face the ground resting on 'cushions of air'. As your hands pass your hips, bend your knees, sink and sit down into your legs – weight 70% in your left leg.

As you raise your arms, breathe in smoothly through your nose. As your arms fall and you sink into the ground, exhale through your nose.

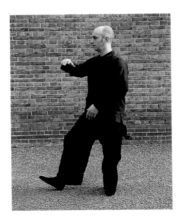

Posture 4: Ward off left

Turn your waist to the right and sink your weight fully into your left leg, lift your right toes away from the ground and allow your right leg to pivot on your right heel. At the same time your right forearm pivots at the elbow until it is parallel to the ground, palm facing down and fingers pointing to the front. Your left arm moves naturally across

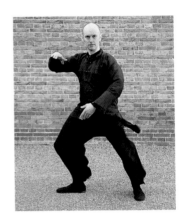

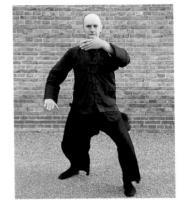

your body, maintaining a soft roundness, until your palm faces the tan tien. Your left arm does not touch your body.

Relax your right foot down and sink your weight into your right leg. As you do this, allow your waist to turn naturally to the left. Do not move your arms. Sink 100% of your weight into your right leg and pick up your relaxed left leg, heel first. Take a short, natural step to the front and place your foot on the ground, heel first.

Gradually shift your weight into your left leg, turning your waist to the left. As you do this, your left arm sweeps upwards until your palm is level with the base of your throat – your arm is rounded with the elbow hanging down slightly, shoulder relaxed. At the same time your right hand falls to a place just below your hip. Keep the arm rounded with the palm resting on a 'cushion of air', fingers pointing to the front. Finish the posture by sitting 70% of your weight down into your left leg and squaring your hips to the front, simultaneously pulling your right toes around to a comfortable position.

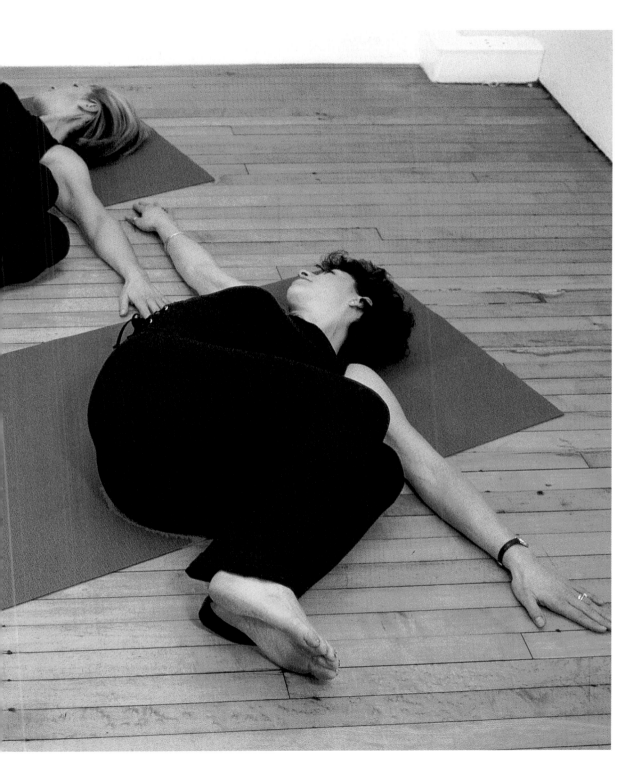

Yoga

The ancient art of yoga is not purely a physical discipline. Yogis view it is as an integrated system affecting mind, body, spirit and heart at many levels: physically (through bones, muscles, organs, circulation, nerves); pranially ('prana' means 'breath' which yogis consider to be the flow of our life-force); psychologically (through our feelings and emotions) and spiritually (through the soul, connecting us to a higher consciousness). The true practice of yoga is not a fast fix.

There are many different disciplines of yoga: Hatha, astanga, bikrum and vinyasa to name a few. Hatha yoga is a gentle practice based on breathing and relaxation, vinyasa and astanga are more pysically challenging, and bikrum yoga is performed in specially heated studios.

The workouts featured in the next few pages provide a taste of yoga to centre mind and body, and to enhance flexibility, strength and balance. Explore the different styles to find one to suit you.

Five postures for beginners

The breath is central to yoga, but correct breathing for beginners takes a little while to establish. A good guideline to start with is to exhale into postures and inhale out of them. Try to complete each breath, inhaling for the same amount of time that you exhale. Take 6–8 breaths in each posture, and make them longer as you become more focused, balanced and established in your practice.

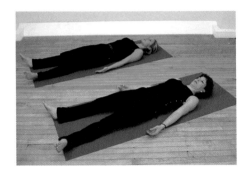

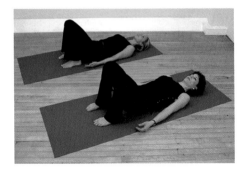

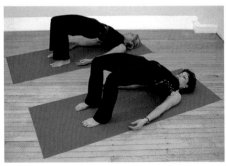

Bridge (Setu Bandha)

Benefits: Improves digestion and strengthens abdominal organs. Relieves back ache and neck strain. Strengthens pelvic floor muscles.

Preparation: Lie flat and exhale as you move your tail bone forward to soften the arch in the lower back, and engage the pelvic floor muscles.

Pose: Draw your heels in towards you. Feet are parallel and there is an even distribution of weight through the mound of the big toe, fanning out to the little toe. Aware of the pelvic floor muscles, draw the abdomen back, contract your buttocks to lift the hips, meanwhile ensure the knees work towards each other and that the inner thighs are strong.

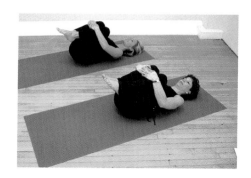
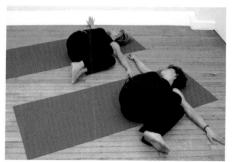
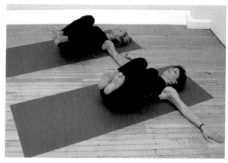
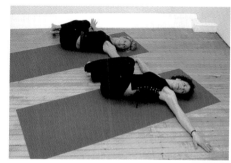

Lying twist (Jathara Parvitasana)

Benefits: Releases tension in the shoulders. Helps with symptoms of constipation and bloatedness. Relieves discomfort in the lower back.

Preparation: Hug the knees in towards the abdomen and clasp the hands under the knees in towards the body to release the hip flexors and improve hip mobility.

Pose: Take your arms out to the side in line with the shoulders. Turn your head to look left and allow the knees to move towards the right elbow. Keep the knees, ankles, calves and thighs together and flex the heels to increase the stretch. If there is weakness in the lower back, make sure the legs are not lifted towards the elbow, but rather in line with or lower than the hip. Repeat on both sides.

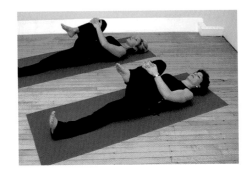
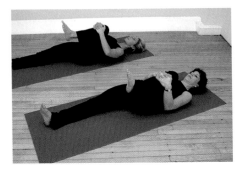
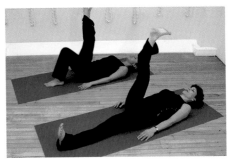
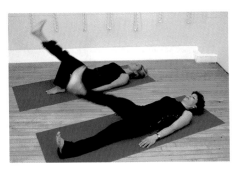

Alternate Leg Raising (Supta Pandangusthasana)

Benefits: Helps to lengthen hamstrings and release tightness and discomfort in the lower back. Helps to align the pelvis, strengthen the knees and can help relieve sciatic pain. It is also beneficial in developing deep abdominal muscles (transverse abdominal muscles).

Preparation: Lower the back on to the mat and hug each leg alternately in towards the body. Ensure you do not tilt the head back – maintain length in the back of the neck.

Pose: Raise the legs alternately – raise the leg as you inhale and lower it as you exhale. Stretch through the hamstrings and lift the knee to engage the quadriceps. Bend the opposite knee if you have lower back discomfort. Do 6 lifts on each leg.

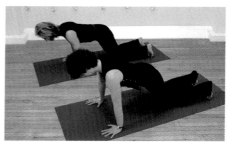
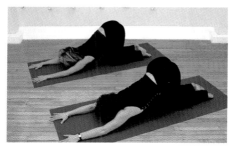

Extended cat pose (hamsasana)

Benefits: Releases tension and tightness in the neck and shoulder area and in the abdominal muscles. Creates a sense of space between the vertebrae, improving posture and the function of the central nervous system.

Preparation: Begin in child's pose and come on to all fours – hands under shoulders and knees under hips. Maintain the knees hip-width apart under the hips to facilitate softness in the abdominal muscles and shoulders.

Pose: Extend the arms forward. Feel the stretch deep into the shoulders and rest either the forehead or chin on your mat as you continue to stretch your arms away from you.

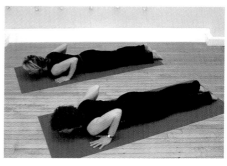
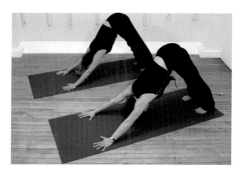

Dog Pose (Aho Mukha Svanasana)

Benefits: Slows the heart rate. Reduces stiffness in the shoulders. Strengthens the ankles and tones the legs. Helps to prevent hot flushes during the menopause.

Preparation: Lie on your stomach. Bring your hands back underneath your shoulders. Ensure that the elbows are tucked in and lift them towards the ceiling. Your forehead rests on your mat.

Pose: Press firmly down into the heels of the hands. Move the tail bone forwards. Move back on to the knees, curl the toes underneath you and sit back on the heels. Raise the hips towards the ceiling. Engage the quadriceps muscles and come on to the balls of your feet. Slowly draw the heels down towards the floor. Work the creases of the elbows towards each other and rotate the upper arms out as you press evenly into the hands and continue to lift upwards from the hands to lengthen down through the heels.

This workout offers more challenging postures. Hold all postures for 8–12 breaths.

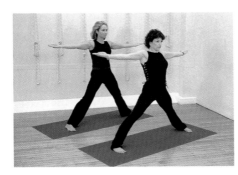
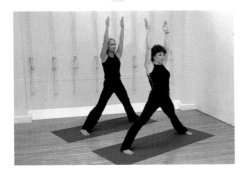
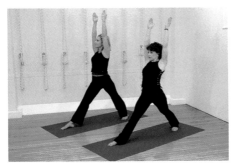
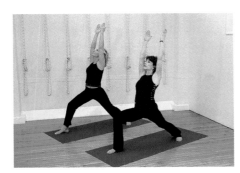

Warrior One (Virabhadrasana 1)

Benefits: Improves digestion and relieves heartburn. Tones abdominal muscles and strengthens the bladder and back muscles.

Preparation: From standing pose (Tadasana), jump the feet approximately 1.2m/4 feet apart. Step or jump the feet apart. Take the arms out to the side and ensure the wrists are in line with the ankles. Extend through the fingertips and rotate the palms upwards. Stretch up towards the ceiling, bringing the palms together. Do not cross the thumbs.

Pose: Turn the right foot 90° and the left foot deep in. Ensure that the hips feel level and the buttocks are in line. Bend the right knee from the right buttock bone. Create a right-angle in the right leg and extend the left leg strongly. Move the weight to the outer edge of the back foot, lifting the inner ankle bone. Ensure the hips remain level and extend up through the spine. Repeat the pose to the left.

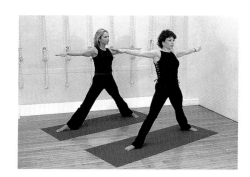
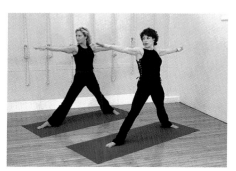
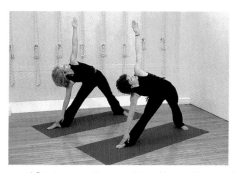
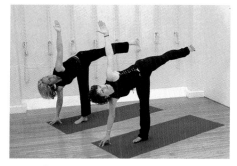

Half Moon Pose (Ardha Chandrasana)

Benefits: Tones the lower spine and nerves connecting the leg muscles. Releases tightness in the sacrum and hamstrings and helps open the muscles of the mid- and upper back.

Preparation: From standing pose (Tadasana), jump the feet approximately 1.2m/4ft apart. Turn the left foot in and the right foot 90°. Press the right heel to the floor and extend the toes towards the ceiling. Tighten the right knee and put the toes back on the floor. Exhale as you extend your torso sideways and bring the right hand (or fingertips) to the floor. Turn your head to look up at your extended left arm (Trikonasana).

Pose: From Trikonasana, bend the right knee and move the right hand 30cm/12in ahead and to the outside of the right foot. Hop the back foot in and establish balance through the supporting hand and standing leg. Push into the big toe and heel of the standing leg and raise the left leg up in line with the foot. Extend through the left heel. Rotate the left hip back and turn to look up at the left hand without straining the neck. Repeat the pose to the left.

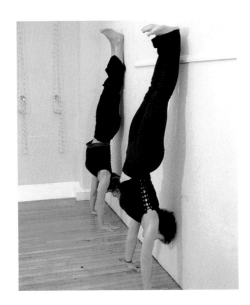

Full Arm Balance (Urdhva Muka Vrksasana)

Benefits: Tones and strengthens the arms. Releases tightness in the shoulder and brings about a feeling of energy and lightness. Improves circulation.

Preparation: Ardho Mukha Svanasana (dog pose). Focus on centring the weight into the middle of the wrists. Ensure the hands are fan-shaped and that the middle finger points forwards. Consciously work the outer calf muscle in, lift through the front of the thighs and extend through the back of the legs. Maintain length in the back of the neck. Broaden the chest and feel the spine lengthening. Move the shoulders back and down towards the waist.

Pose: Place the hands shoulder-width apart with the fingertips a few centimetres from the wall. Imagine pushing the floor away with your arms. Kick up into a handstand one leg at a time. Balance for as long as possible, gaze at a point on the floor and extend from the lower back up to the heels.

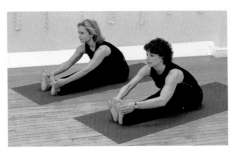 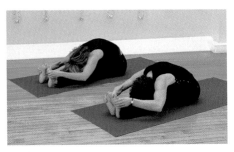

Forward bend (Paschimottanasana)

Benefits: Rests the heart and the adrenal glands. Improves digestive and liver functions. Helps the entire reproductive system.

Preparation: Start in Dandasana and lift flesh away from the buttocks. Stretch your arms so that you hold the outer edges of the feet. Press thighs down to the floor to stretch more effectively. Broaden the front of the body.

Pose: Hold around the soles of the feet and interlock the fingers or hold the wrist. Lift the torso further and bend forwards from the lower back. Stretch equally from both sides of the waist. Place the forehead on the knees and move it towards the shins. Widen the elbows to open the chest further.

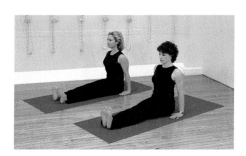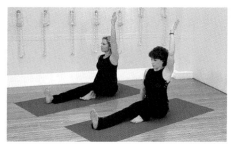

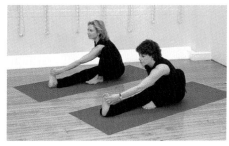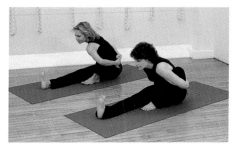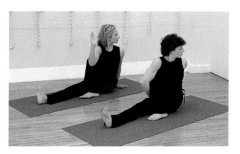

Sitting Twist (marichyasana C)

Benefits: Tones and massages the abdominal organs. Improves the liver, intestinal and kidney function. Reduces the waistline. Relieves back ache.

Preparation: Sit in Dandasana (upright with the right leg out in front of you and the sole of the left foot on the floor about one hand space from the left inner thigh). Reach forwards with the left hand inside the left knee and wrap the left hand back around the left shin. The right palm faces away from the body and the left arm rotates around to join the right, behind the back.

Pose: Leg position as above. Exhale as you lift your spine and turn the torso 90° to the left. Move the right shoulder forwards and place the right elbow over the left knee. Allow weight into the left hand behind you. Push into left ankle and rotate further to the left, turning from the waist. Take your left hand behind your back and join hands, working towards holding the wrist. (Try the modified version – my position, above – if you are unable to bind your hands behind your back.) Repeat this pose on the other side.

Pilates

Pilates is a form of exercise designed by Joseph Pilates to strengthen and lengthen dancers' muscles. It specifically works on the deep core stability muscles to reduce back pain, improve posture and realign the body.

Mat pilates classes are generally popular in health clubs. Using small props and mats, these classes use the basic pilates techniques but without the specialist equipment, such as reformer beds, pilates carriages and chair equipment, found in professional pilates studios.

In the workouts that follow, you should aim to do 1 set of 8 repetitions of each in the sequence

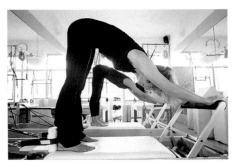 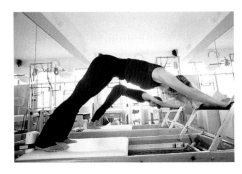

Elephant

What it does: Flattens and strengthens the abdominals, lengthens the hamstrings and strengthens the shoulder girdle.

What you do: Place the feet flat, heels against the Pilates carriage with the shoulders relaxed and the back rounded in flexion, ribs pulled in and hands holding the foot bar. Keep the arms long and avoid hyper-extending the elbows by keeping the elbows slightly soft. Using the legs and abdominals, push the carriage out. Use your arms to stabilize your body and not push the carriage away. Return the carriage forwards using the abdominals and hamstrings and pull in your ribs as you remain in a C-curve.

Top Tip: Don't hyper-extend the knees and elbows!

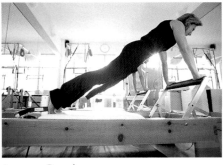 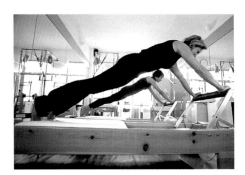

Long Back

What it does: Tones the abdominals, gluteals and hamstrings.

What you do: Place the heels of the hands on the foot bar with the balls of the feet and heels lifted against the shoulder rests. Keep the spine neutral, pelvis level and legs long, parallel and together. Your shoulder blades need to be down to keep the shoulder girdle in place. Press the carriage out, using abdominals and legs. Maintain your torso in a dart position and return the carriage and body forwards to the start position.

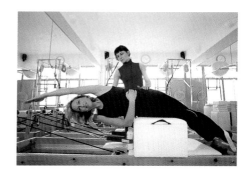
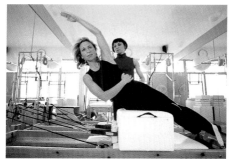

Side Over Sitting On Box

What it does: Strengthens the obliques, lower back muscles and shoulder-girdle muscles.

What you do: Sit sideways on the box with one foot hooked under the foot strap. Keep a neutral spine and pelvis. Lengthen up through the body and bend the torso sideways towards the floor. Come up to vertical and lengthen up and sideways over towards the foot bar. Repeat on the other side.

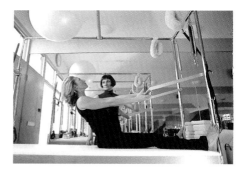
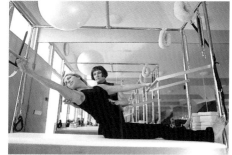

Back Extension With Rotation

What it does: Flattens the abdominals and gluteals, and strengthens the shoulder girdle.

What you do: Roll down on to the sit bones and contract your abdominals to stay in a C-curve. Keep the shoulder blades down and back. Diagonally reach the arm back, and stabilize with the shoulder blade to keep the neck long. Extend the upper back slightly as you reach back over your head and take the bar. Repeat on the other side.

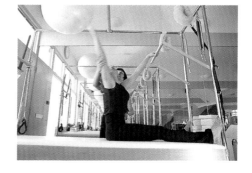
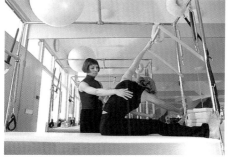

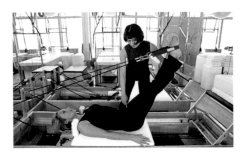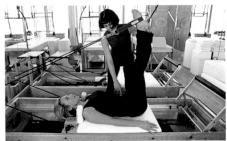

Short Spinal

What it does: Strengthens and flattens the abdominals. Tones gluteals, hamstrings and inner thighs.

What you do: Lie face-up on the carriage. Draw your lower spine to the carriage. Place your feet in the 2 straps, lengthen your legs and contract in your inner thighs to keep the legs together. Roll up on to the shoulder girdle, peeling each vertebra using your abdominals. Drop the knees towards the shoulders. Remain in a curved position as you roll the tail back towards the foot bar, keeping the legs bent. Extend the legs and go back to the start position.

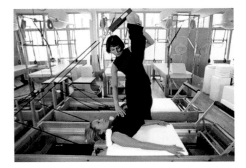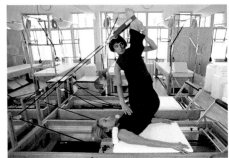

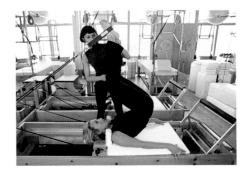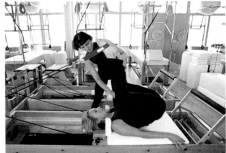

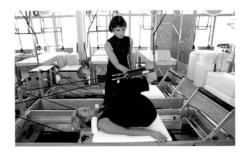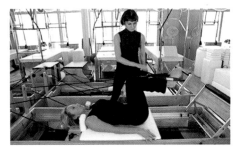

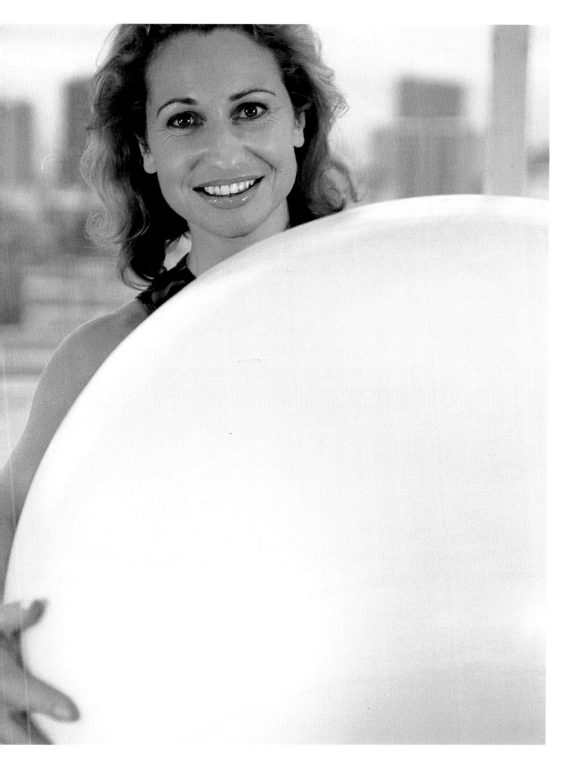

Balance and stability work

Balance work should play an important part in the fitness programme of any individual. Like flexibility work, it can directly affect the quality of day-to-day living and reduce your risk of injury through falls. Balance work uses visual information as well as the neurological activation of specific muscles. Balance work is not just about standing on one leg, effective balance relies on flexibility, strength of the core trunk muscles and good muscle co-ordination.

This workout has been designed to address all these areas. To ensure the best results, focus on your technique and avoid rushing.

Workout: Improve Your Stability and Balance

Body Kit
Swiss Exercise ball

Mat

The Workout
Stability Bridge x 4

Stability Bridge With Ball x 4

Opposite Arm and Leg Reach x 8 (see page 101)

Same Arm, Same Leg Reach x 8

Eagle Pose x 1 right and left

Single Leg Balance x 1 right and left

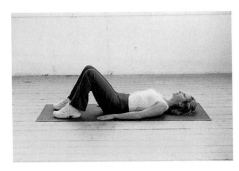 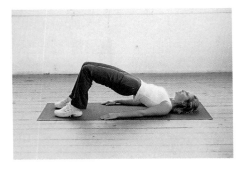

Stability Bridge

What it does: Improves the stability of the trunk muscles of the back and the abdominals.

What you do: Lie on your back, heels and toes touching the floor, arms at your sides. With a neutral spine, use your hip, thigh and trunk muscles to lift your pelvis until your body forms one line from your shoulders to your knees. Slowly lower yourself to the starting position.

How many? 4–10

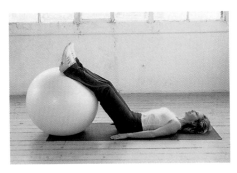 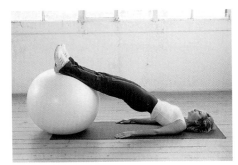 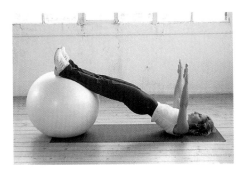

Stability Bridge With Ball

What it does: This is a more challenging exercise designed to strengthen the core stability muscles of the torso, as well as the hamstrings, buttocks and quadriceps.

What you do: Lie on your back, heels on top of an exercise ball, knees slightly bent, arms at your sides. Do the same bridge exercise as above. Maintain your balance by pressing your heels down into the ball. Slowly lower to the starting position.

How many? 4–10

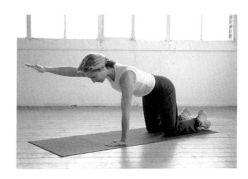
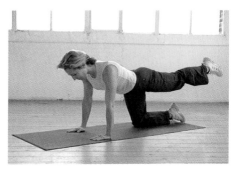
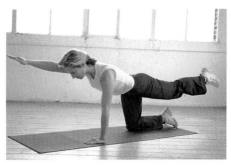
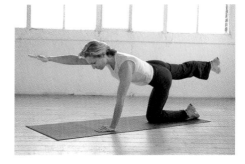

Same Arm, Same Leg Reach

What it does: This is a challenging exercise that encourages whole body balance through the contraction of the abdominal muscles and spine extensors.

What you do: On all fours, place your wrists under your shoulders and your knees under your hips. Establish a neutral spine and contract your abdominals. Slowly stretch your right arm and right leg away from the floor, bringing them level with your torso. Aim to hold for a count of 8 and slowly lower down. Repeat with the left arm and left leg. An easier version entails reaching one limb at a time and building up to lifting both limbs at the same time.

How many? 8

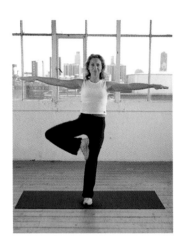

Eagle Pose

What it does: This posture comes from yoga. It will strengthen the muscles of the foot and ankle, which are crucial to help maintain balance – especially as we get older.

What you do: Stand with good posture. Draw your weight on to your left leg, lift the right leg and place the sole of the foot on the inside of the inner left thigh. Apply equal pressure to both the foot and the inner thigh – this will help you keep your balance. Lift the arms out to the sides, and focus on keeping as still as possible. Hold for up to 30 seconds. Repeat on the other side. To make this more more challenging, try shutting your eyes

How many? Up to 4 on each side

Top Tip: Contracting up through the pelvic floor will help your balance.

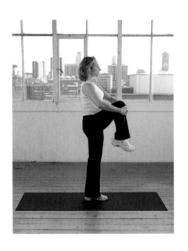

Single Leg Balance

What it does: Shutting your eyes as you try to balance encourages proprioceptive nerve communication between the brain and the muscles.

What you do: Stand with good posture. Draw your weight on to one leg and lift your knee in to your chest. Extend up through the spine and, when you feel balanced, challenge yourself to shut your eyes. Feel how the foot muscles work hard to stabilize it. Try to hold for 30 seconds.

How many? Up to 4 on each side

Top Tip: You may wish to have a chair near you to help you get your balance as you start.

Targeted Muscle Group: Hamstrings

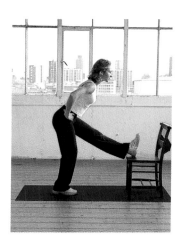

Standing Hamstring

What you do: Stand with good posture. Extend one leg out in front of you. Bend the back knee and flex forwards from the hips. Make sure you contract your abdominals as you extend forwards. Lift up out of the hips and check they are level. To help you, imagine you need to balance a glass of water on each side of your lower back.

How long? Hold for up to 30 seconds

Top Tip: To improve the stretch, lift your leg and rest it on a bench, low step or chair.

Top tip

Muscles attach to the bone at different sites, so to stretch effectively, it is a good idea to perform various positions on both sides. Do experiment with the stretches shown and feel the difference for yourself.

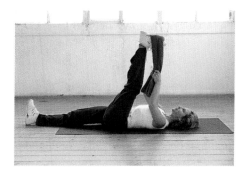

Lying Hamstring

What you do: Lie on your back and establish neutral posture. Slowly draw one leg in to your chest and extend the leg at the knee. Keep the hips down on the floor and the upper body relaxed. You can hold on to the thigh and calf for support.

How long? Hold for up to 30 seconds

Top Tip: Use a towel to help you support the leg.

Targeted Muscle Group: Quadriceps

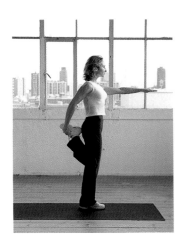

Standing Quad

What you do: Stand with good posture. Lift one leg, bending at the knee, holding the laces of your shoe in your hand. Keep the knees together. Gently press your hips forwards as you extend up through your spine.

How long? Hold for 10–15 seconds. Repeat on the other side.

Top Tip: If you have limited flexibility, rest your foot on a chair and press your hips forward.

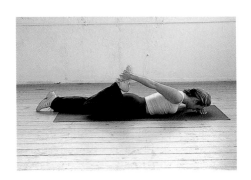

Lying Quad

What you do: Lie face-down on the floor. Contract your abdominals to support your spine. Bend your leg at the knee, bringing your foot to your bottom, and reach back with the hand on the same side as the lifted leg to hold on to the ankle or shoe laces. Keep the knees together.

How long? Hold for 10–15 seconds. Repeat on the other side.

Top Tip: Press the hips into the floor to increase the stretch.

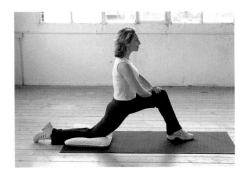

Standing Hip Flexor

What you do: Come into a lunge position. Make sure your front knee is over your ankle and your knee is in line with your second toe. Extend the back leg, pressing the pelvis down to the floor. Hold the laces of your shoe, or, if you need support, hang on to a chair or door.

How long? Hold for 10–15 seconds

Pilates Saw

What you do: Sit with good posture, legs open. Extend up through the spine and lift the arms out to the sides, level with the shoulders. Keep both hips on the floor as you pivot your upper body towards one side. Extend forwards with your arms as you reach over your extended leg. Keep lifted from the pelvis, with abdominals contracted.

How long? This is an active stretch with no holding phase.

Top Tip: This is a challenging stretch, which you may feel in your lower back and inner thighs. Bend the legs in to reduce the intensity of the stretch.

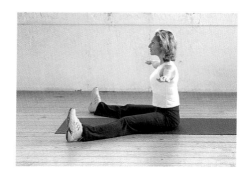 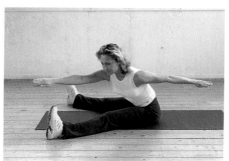

Targeted Muscle Group: Gluteals

Seated Gluteal Stretch

What you do: Sit on a chair with good posture. Place your arms beside you with your hands supporting your body on the chair. Your fingers should be pointing towards your toes. Lift one leg and place that ankle on the other knee. Support your body weight in your hands and lift yourself off the chair, slowly lowering yourself towards the floor. You should feel a deep stretch on the buttock of the crossed leg.

How long? Hold for 10–15 seconds

Top Tip: If you suffer from knee pain you are advised to do the lying gluteal stretch instead.

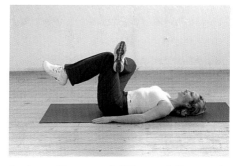

Lying Crossed Gluteal Stretch

What you do: This is a variation on the Seated Gluteal Stretch, as it is performed in a lying-down position.

How long? Hold for 10–15 seconds

Top Tip: If you rest your supporting leg against a wall, you can reduce tension in your upper shoulders.

Lying Gluteal Stretch

What you do: Lie on your back. Establish neutral posture. Extend one leg down to the floor and draw the other knee in to the chest, holding it behind the knee cap. Make sure you establish your abdominal contraction to stretch the gluteals effectively.

How long? Hold for 10–15 seconds.

Targeted Body Part: Lower legs

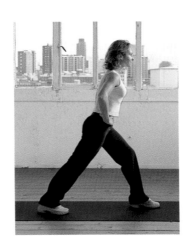

Standing Calf Stretch

What you do: Stand with good posture. Take a large step backwards, making sure both feet are facing forwards. Keep the front knee over the ankle and check the middle of the knee cap is in line with the second toe. Press the back heel down to the floor. Make sure the body makes a straight line from the top of your head to your back foot. Repeat with the other leg.

How long: Hold for 10–15 seconds

Top Tip: Push against a wall for extra support and contract your gluteals to increase the stretch. To stretch more into the lower calf, bring the back leg in a little and bend it at the knee.

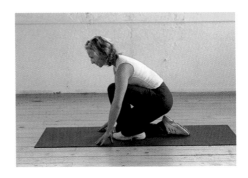

Achilles Stretch

What you do: Crouch down to place one foot on the ground and rest the other knee on the floor beside the flat foot. Keep the foot flat on the floor and lean forward over your knee until you feel a stretch on the Achilles of that foot. Repeat with the other leg.

How long? Hold for 10–15 seconds

Top Tip: The achilles tendon can be quite stiff. Perform this stretch, together with the single leg balance (see page 128), to improve your range of motion.

Targeted Muscle Group: Outer Thighs

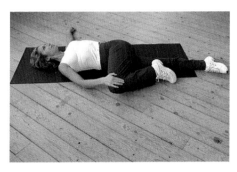 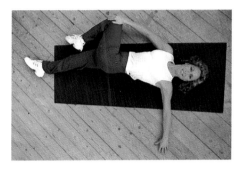 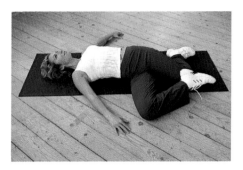

Lying Spine Twist

What you do: Lie on the floor face-up with your legs extended flat out. Lift your left knee towards the chest and gently ease it across the right side of your body, supporting it with the right hand. As far as possible keep the knee at 90° to the torso. You are aiming to get the inside of the left knee the floor on you right side. Breathe in a controlled manner and do only what is comfortable for you. Contract the abdominals and release your leg to the floor. Repeat on the other leg.

How long? Hold for 10–30 seconds

Top Tip: To increase the stretch, place one foot on the opposing knee and gently press down.

Targeted Muscle Group: Inner Thighs

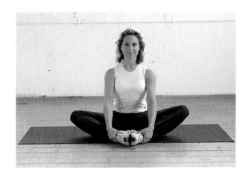

Inner Thigh Stretch

What you do: Sit with good posture, place the soles of your feet together and allow the knees to drop open. Gently press the knees to the floor.

How long? Hold for 10–15 seconds

Top Tip: To develop this position, open the legs to the sides, and slowly ease the body forwards.

Targeted Body Part: Full Body

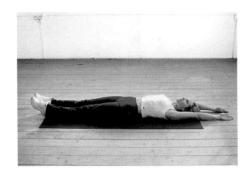

Lying Full Body Stretch

What you do: Lie on the floor face-up. Extend your arms above your head. Gently stretch and lengthen through the whole body from your fingertips to your toes. Your lower back may come gently off the floor. Breathe gently. Slowly bring your arms down by your sides.

How long? Hold for up to 30 seconds

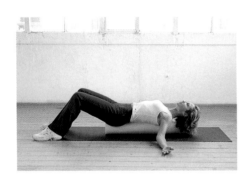

Foam Roller Stretch

What you do: Lie on a Pilates foam roller face-up. Place the arms a little distance away from the body with the palms up.

How long? Hold for up to 30 seconds.

Top Tip: This is a great position to relax in and practise your meditation exercise (see page 98).

Targeted Body Part: Upper Body

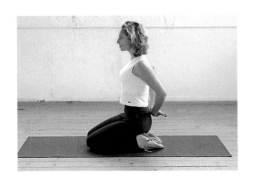

Chest Stretch

What you do: Stand or kneel with good posture and lift your arms out to the sides and behind. Keep the shoulders down as you hold on to your wrists. Check the back stays in a neutral position as you draw your hands together.

How long? Hold for 10–15 seconds

Top Tip: You can isolate one chest muscle by placing the palm down against a wall and leaning away from your hand.

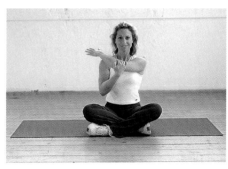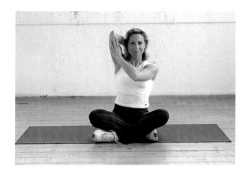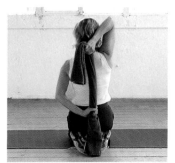

Seated Triceps Stretch

What you do: Sit with good posture. Lift one arm above the head and drop the palm of the hand behind the head between the shoulder blades. Lift the other arm and support the stretching arm either by pressing gently from the front on the soft fleshy part of the arm or above on the elbow. This stretch can also be performed standing.

How long? Hold for 10–15 seconds

Top Tip: If you have limited shoulder mobility, holding a towel avoids discomfort by helping to ease the shoulder joint.

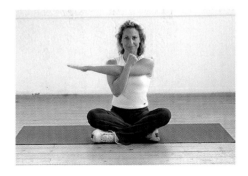

Seated Deltoid Stretch

What you do: Sit with good posture. Extend one arm out in front of you and cross it in front of the mid-line of the body. Keep both shoulders facing forward. Support the stretching arm on the fleshy part of the forearm.

How long? Hold for 10–15 seconds

All Fours Trapezius Stretch

What you do: On all fours, wrists under shoulders and knees under hips, slide one hand, palm upwards, between your knee and arm, away from the body. Gently allow the shoulder of the extended arm to relax and open. You should feel a gentle opening behind the shoulders.

How long? Hold for 10–15 seconds

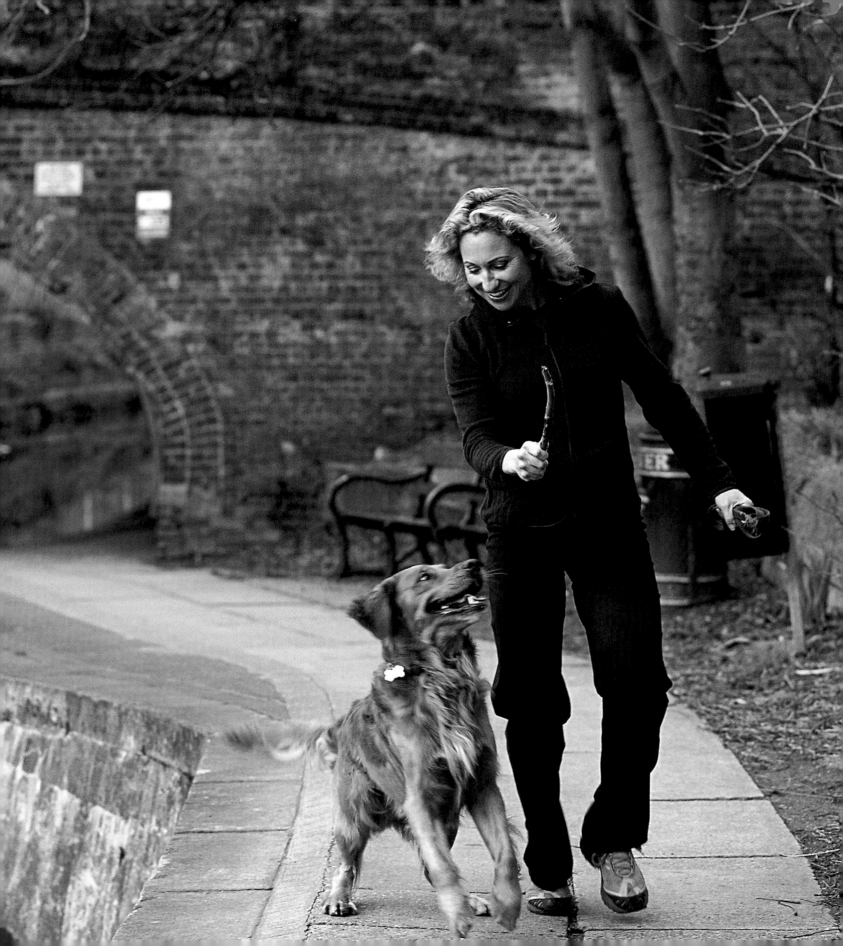

exercise and lifestyle

We may want to fit exercise into our schedules, but all too often our busy lifestyles prevent us from being as active as we would like. The weeks go by, the months add up and before we know it we have entered another decade. Just as our lives and lifestyles evolve, so too do our bodies change. What we need to do to keep ourselves fit and healthy in our youth is quite different from the requirements of a more mature body. But whatever your age or the challenges life throws at you, there are simple and effective opportunities to be active!

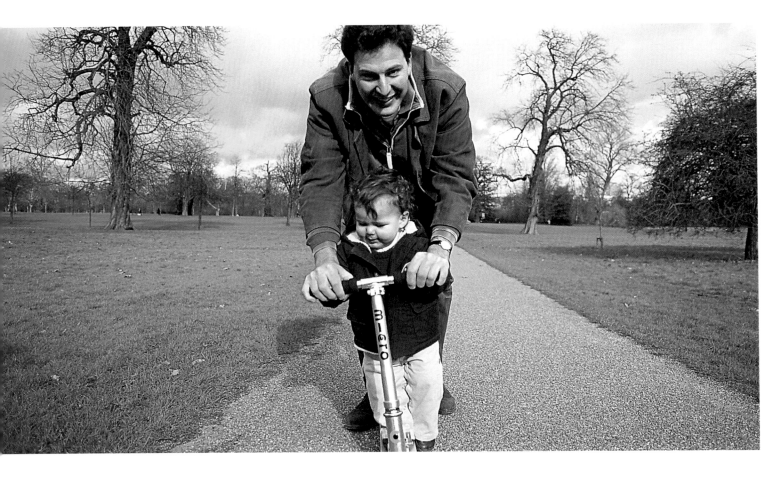

We are now less active than our parents were, and as a result heart disease, cancers, diabetes and osteoporosis are more prevalent than ever before. Making exercise fit into our lifestyle and life-stages represents a huge challenge, but whether you are 7 or 70, there are still small things you can do to improve your health, fitness and body shape, wherever you are, whatever your motivation and whatever you want to achieve.

Health organisations have set out the following simple guidelines to promote health and longevity:

- **Get adequate sleep**
- **Eat a good breakfast**
- **Eat regular meal and avoid snacks**
- **Control your weight**
- **Abstain from smoking**
- **Drink moderately**
- **Exercise regularly**

However, the pace and stresses of life often prevent us from following these simple recommendations. Stress levels can contribute to poor eating habits, smoking and disturbed sleep patterns. Erratic eating disrupts regular meals and

weight control, and long working hours and sedentary lifestyles hamper our attempts to exercise regularly.

With fitness awareness on the rise, many parents now know that children need activity just as much as adults do. The problem is discovering just what kind of exercise is appropriate for bodies that are still growing, as there are significant physiological differences between children and adults in both the respiratory and cardiovascular systems. A child's body is not just a smaller version of ours.

children

Children have lower stroke volumes and higher heart rates than adults at all exercise intensities. In addition, both children and adolescents have higher maximum heart rates than adults, so methods for estimating maximum heart rates (as detailed in Chapter 2) cannot be used for children or for adolescents until their late teens. Children and teenagers do not sweat as much as adults during exercise, as their sweat glands do not become fully effective until late in adolescence. This means that, when exercising in extreme cold or heat, they do not acclimatize so well and are more prone to heat exhaustion. Couple this with the fact that children do not have an effective thirst mechanism, and you have an age group which is susceptible to dehydration and heat exhaustion. Make sure your children drink plenty of fluids before, during and after exercise, as thirst may not be an accurate indicator of their requirements. (For tips on hydration, see page 219.)

Ages 2–8

The focus of exercise in early childhood should be on the development of basic movement skills such as running, balancing, jumping and co-ordination. Exercise should centre around making movement fun. Yoga-style movements can be a great way for children to explore their bodies, incorporate all the movement skills and boost their physical self-confidence.

Playing with animal shapes and noises in the Yoga Bug Postures (see page 140) brings an element of fun to this physical workout. And while the Brain Gym for Kids (page 142) is highly effective for training the brain, the beauty of it is that your children won't even notice!

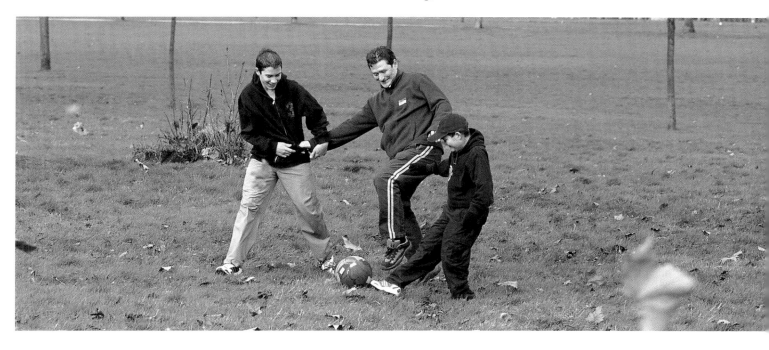

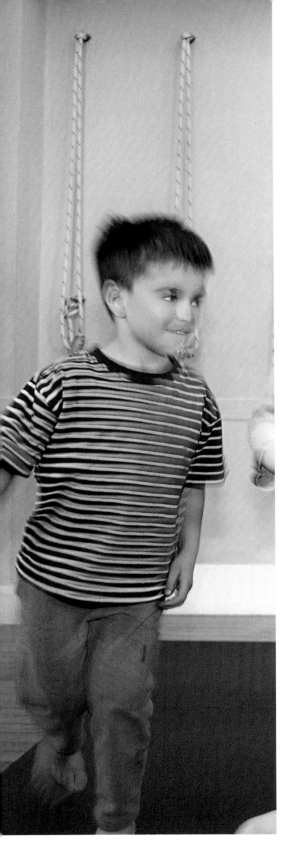

Yoga Bugs™ Workout

These postures are ideally suited to children aged between 3 and 8 years. There are no rules stipulating how long the postures should be held, or how many repetitions to do: the best guideline is for as long as the child is comfortable and having fun.

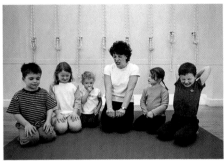

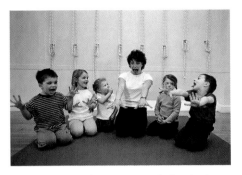

Lion

What it does: Helps you let go of any bad things in your head or worries on your mind. Gives you a feeling of wanting to jump up and feel happy or say sorry to people who you might have made sad.

What you do: Sit back on your heels with your hands flat on your thighs. Close your eyes and take a few long, slow breaths. Move from the heels to the knees and extend your arms fiercely out in front of you. Open your eyes wide, open your mouth and stick out your tongue. Let out a loud 'h-a-a' sound, feeling as if you are king of the jungle.

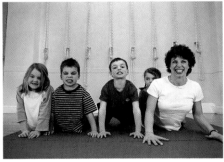

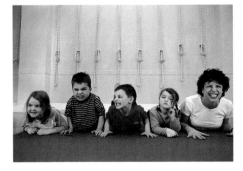

Snake

What it does: Makes your arms and back feel very strong. Gives your tummy a nice stretch and helps you to stand very tall.

What you do: Lie on your tummy and rest your head on your arms. Stretch your toes away from you and make your thighs feel very strong. Bring your hands back underneath your shoulders and let your elbows point to the ceiling. Push your bottom down to the floor, push down into your hands and lift your head and body off the floor, keeping your elbows bent. Make a loud hissing sound and a very mean face.

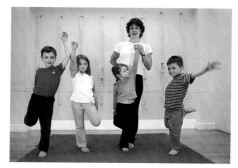

Tree

What it does: This helps you to be better at listening and understanding things. It's a very good balance and makes your legs stronger so you can run even faster.

What you do: Stand on both feet like a tall soldier. Make one leg feel very heavy and the other feel light. Bring the light leg up and hold onto your foot while you stand strongly on the heavy leg. When you feel tall and steady as a tree, stretch your free hand up above you to be a really tall and strong tree.

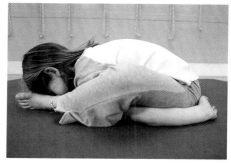

Tortoise

What it does: Helps your hips to move in all the directions you need them to. Gives your back a lovely stretch and makes you feel quiet, still and slow like a tortoise.

What you do: Sit on your bottom and bring your feet and legs out in front of you. Stretch forward and bring your feet together so that the bits that you stand on are touching. Bring your head towards your feet. Take your arms underneath your legs and turn them so that you try to bring your hands together behind your back. Little people are good at this – usually better than grown-ups.

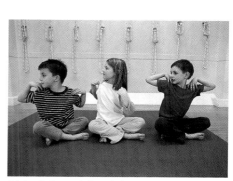

Washing Machine

What it does: Helps to stop you getting a sore neck and back like mummy or daddy sometimes gets and makes you very good at sitting up straight.

What you do: Sit with your legs crossed and your knees

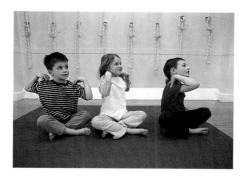

bent. Put your hands on your shoulders and have your elbows out to the sides. Move your elbows around in big circles and imagine that you are washing all the grubby bits and marks out of your clothes.

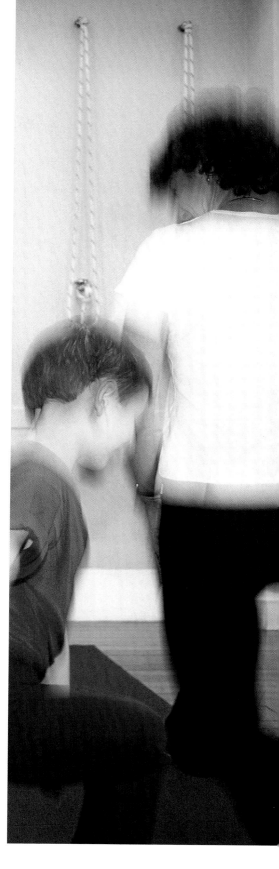

Brain Gym™ for Kids

We may encourage physical exercise, but do we ever give our children's brains a good workout? Brain Gym™ aims to do just that. The theory behind it is to use movement to stimulate neurological pathways and help both sides of the brain to work together. Repeated studies have found that 80% of children with learning difficulties have trouble integrating their left and right brain hemispheres.

The left hemisphere of the brain controls the right side of the body and deals with academic functions such as arithmetic and language. The right side controls the body's left side and is responsible for our emotions and understanding.

The Brain Gym™ exercises were developed by a Californian educationalist, Dr Paul Dennison, in the late 1960s. Severely dyslexic himself, he was intrigued by the connection between physical activity and learning ability. The exercises have growing support and Brain Gym teachers report an improvement in their students' reading, writing and maths as well as memory, concentration and general co-ordination.

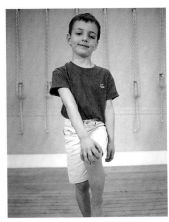

Cross Crawl

What it does: Helps with reading, writing, listening, memory and co-ordination.

What you do: While standing, lift your right knee and touch it with your left hand, then lift your left knee and touch it with your right hand.

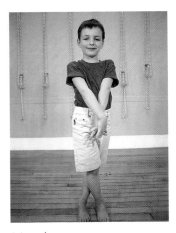

Hook-up

What it does: Helps with stress, self-esteem and listening.

What you do: While sitting or standing, cross one ankle over the other. Cross one wrist (the same side as the ankle) over the other and touch your palms together,

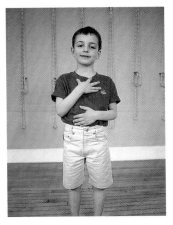

Brain Button

What it does: Aids clear thinking, reading and focus.

What you do: Make a U-shape with the thumb and index finger of one hand, place it in the centre of your chest. Gently rub this acupressure point for 30 seconds and place your other hand over your navel. Change hands and repeat.

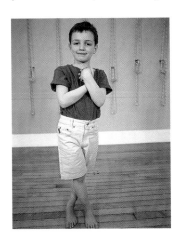

thumbs downwards. Interlace your fingers and draw your hands up towards your chest. Rest your tongue on the roof of your mouth so your jaw relaxes. Stay like this for 1 minute, eyes closed, breathing deeply. Then change your feet and hands around and cross them the other way.

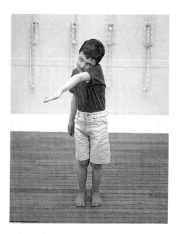

Elephant

What it does: Helps with hand-eye co-ordination and focus.

What you do: Place your left ear on your left shoulder, extend your left arm and, with your knees relaxed, use your outstretched hand to draw a lying-down figure '8', starting from the middle and moving the hands upwards to draw the left 'bulge' of the 8 first. Look down your arm at your hand while you are doing it. Switch arms after 3–5 signs.

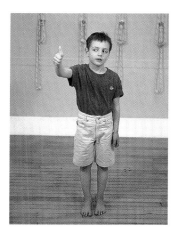

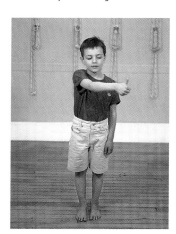

Lazy Eight

What it does: Helps with reading, writing and hand-eye co-ordination.

What you do: Extend one arm in front. With the thumb pointing upwards, slowly and smoothly trace a large figure '8' on its side in the air. Keep your neck relaxed and your head upright, moving only slightly as you focus on your thumb and follow it round. Change arms.

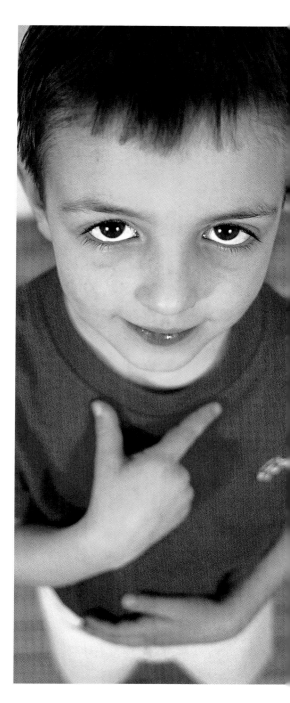

Ages 9–12

This is usually a time when children are becoming more aware of their bodies. Girls especially may be approaching puberty and this will heighten their self-awareness. In addition work pressures at school will also be changing, more time will be spent on computers and less time allocated to physical movement. To avoid long periods of inactivity, schedule activity zones and technology-free zones with your family at the weekends. Encourage active pursuits such as rollerblading, football and skipping. Playful gizmos such as scooters and hoops can act as useful motivators to keep this age group interested in activity.

Teen years

During the teen years, focus on game-type activities which entertain as well as develop co-ordination. Older teens may be ready to concentrate on specific body areas and have exercise and physical-activity goals. They will be more aware of their bodies and may share adult concerns about weight loss and body shape. However, care needs to be taken to present a healthy message of moderate physical activity and not an obsession with body shape and size which can distort the teenager's perception of their body image. In addition, this age group may be more self-conscious and therefore more receptive to exercise if the sexes are separated.

Teenagers need cardiovascular conditioning to improve the health of heart and lungs and to stimulate bone plate loading (a process whereby the bone tissue is encouraged to become denser and stronger). Establishing the exercise habit as part of an active lifestyle is important, and parents need to look to themselves as pivotal role models in their children's attitude to activity. Group aerobics, team sports and yoga can all play a role in adolescent activity. School team sports such as basketball, soccer and hockey also provide an important opportunity for social interaction. However, if your children are naturally sporty, do encourage them to be active outside their sports.

Building in physical-activity habits that will stay with them for life is vitally important for long-term health. Studies have shown that being active in your younger years has no protective effect against heart disease and cancers if the physical activity is not maintained.

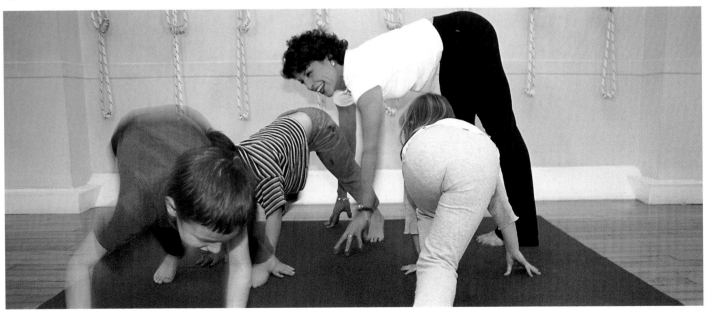

Pregnancy

With sound advice, mums-to-be can continue (or even begin) to exercise during pregnancy. The American College of Obstetricians and Gynaecologists (ACOG) states that pregnant women can reap the health benefits associated with regular, mild to moderate exercise, providing that there are no complications with the pregnancy. Many women have found that regular exercise during pregnancy offsets the physiological changes the body is going through, as well as the psychological changes and inevitable weight gain.

How exercise can help

Exercise increases your cardiovascular stamina so that you can cope more easily with the demands of pregnancy. It can help to reduce minor related ailments such as varicose veins, constipation and stiffness. The Royal College of Midwives encourages a balanced exercise programme to improve posture and body awareness – this is essential as your centre of gravity shifts with the inevitable upward and outward change in your body. Exercising your pelvic floor muscles and abdominal wall muscles regularly will help them to regain strength and

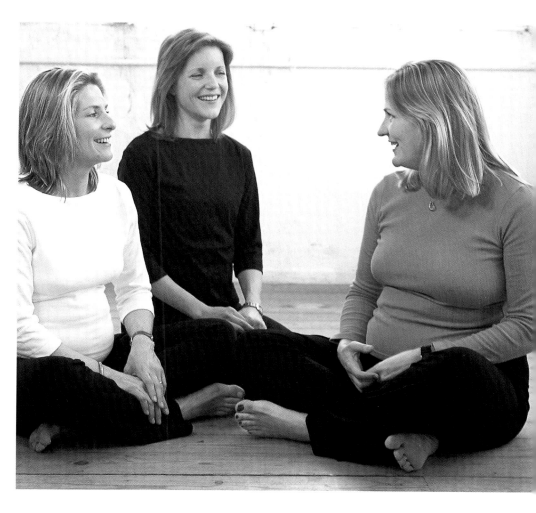

tone more quickly after delivery.

Exercising safely

The ACOG have made the following recommendations for women who are enjoying a healthy pregnancy:

1. **Avoid exercise in the supine position (lying on your back) after the first trimester. This position is associated with decreased cardiac output in most pregnant women and reduces blood flow to your baby. As a consequence standard abdominal curl**

exercises need to be adjusted to maintain abdominal strength as the foetus continues to grow (see pages 147–9 for abdominal exercises).

2. **Avoid prolonged periods of motionless standing.**

3. **Modify your exercise intensity so that you always work within your comfort zone. The ACOG recommends a rate of perceived exertion (see page 41) of 13 – somewhat hard. Reduced oxygen levels in the blood during aerobic activity will make pre-pregnancy aerobic activities more demanding. STOP if you feel tired, dizzy or nauseous, and remember that you should be able to hold a conversation as you are exercising. Non-weight-bearing activity such as swimming or cycling can be particularly enjoyable for pregnant mums-to-be and will minimize the risk of injury.**

4. **Avoid raising body temperature excessively, particularly in the first trimester, as this could be harmful to the development of the baby.**

5. **Isometric exercises (where the muscle is held in one position whilst contracting) should be avoided, as these may increase blood pressure. Abdominal and pelvic floor exercises are, however, the exceptions.**

6. **Pregnancy requires an extra 300 calories per day for normal metabolic activity to be maintained. So women who exercise should pay extra attention to their diet.**

7. **Stay well hydrated, wear appropriate clothing and exercise in an environment that is well ventilated.**

Make sure you check with your GP, midwife or obstetrician before exercising. The benefits of exercise are there to be enjoyed by all, but if any risk factors exist, modifications to your exercise programme are needed. Avoid exercise if you have any of the following conditions:

- **Pregnancy-induced hypertension**
- **Pre-term rupture of membranes**
- **Pre-term labour during former pregnancy**
- **Incompetent cervix**
- **Persistent second- or third-trimester bleeding**
- **Intrauterine growth retardation**

Even though there is no close link between exercise and miscarriage, women with a history of miscarriage should seek medical advice before exercising. Women with certain other medical conditions such as a hyperactive thyroid, chronic hypertension, or cardiac, vascular or pulmonary disease, should be assessed medically to establish an appropriate exercise programme.

Modifying existing routines

Women who are already regular exercisers when they become pregnant are advised not to try to improve their fitness during their pregnancy. The body is already going through significant changes without the additional physiological challenge of a serious training regime. Instead your exercise should be modified so that you can maintain and enjoy your fitness and improve areas of your body that require special attention during this time of change.

Keep high-impact and jerky movements to a minimum. Change from running to power-walking, for example, and switch from high-impact to low-impact aerobics or swimming.

If weight-training, keep the weight light and repetitions moderate.

Reduce the duration of held stretches so that you don't over-extend your joints or cause injury. The increased production of the hormone relaxin can destabilize some joints.

Useful tips

- **Wear a supportive bra and correct foot wear (see Clothing Guidelines, page 236).**
- **Sip water throughout the exercise session to avoid over-heating.**
- **Avoid exercising on an empty stomach.**
- **Always exercise with controlled movements.**

Pregnancy – three trimesters, three exercises

As your baby grows inside you, your centre of gravity changes, your posture is challenged and your abdominal muscles are stretched. You can still train these muscles throughout your pregnancy, however some adaptations are required to safeguard your body. Strong abdominals will help you support your spine, push during delivery and reclaim your shape after your baby is born.

First Trimester

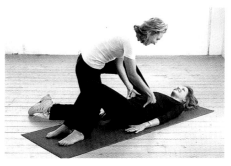

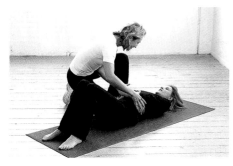

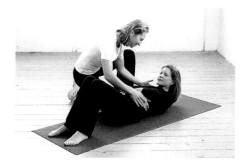

Abdominal Curl With Arm Support

What it does: Supports the rectus abdominal wall.

What you do: Lie on your back, as for a regular abdominal curl. Establish trunk tension and cross your arms over the abdominals, holding lightly on to the sides of your waist.

Curl up, leading from the breastbone, drawing the arms around the waist to support the abdominal wall as you curl. Breathe smoothly. Slowly lower down.

How many? 12–16

The Kegal exercise

This exercise trains the pelvic floor muscles which form a hammock-like structure across the base of the urinary passage. To identify them, imagine you are sitting on the toilet and you need to stop your urine flow. The muscles you contract to do this are the pelvic floor muscles. Please note that it is not advisable to do this in practice as as it can contribute to infection. Instead, focus on drawing the muscles up inside your body while keeping your buttocks relaxed. Perform slow, gradual movements, contracting for a count of 10 and then releasing, followed by a faster action, contracting and realeasing every 2 seconds.

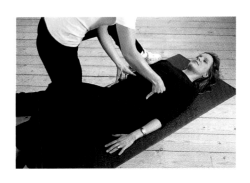

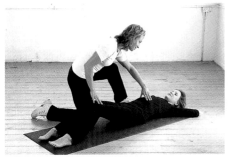

Hip Hitch

What it does: Maintains the tone of the oblique muscles.

What you do: Lie on your back as above, hands by your sides. Keep the tailbone on the floor as you hitch your right hip towards your right ribs. At the same time stretch your right hand to your toes.

How many? 12–16

Pelvic Tilt

What it does: Encourages the strength of the lower abdominal transverse muscle.

What you do: Lie on the floor as above. Establish trunk tension and then draw the pelvic bone off the floor and towards the breastbone. Focus on scooping the abdominal wall flat to the floor as you lift. Release down.

How many? 12–16

Second Trimester

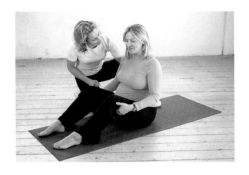

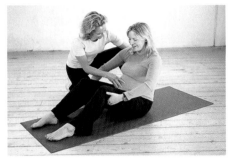

Seated Abdominal Tuck

What it does: Strengthens the abdominal wall.

What you do: Sit upright on the floor, knees bent and feet flat, hands resting lightly behind the thighs. Slowly lean back, contracting your abdominals and tilting your tailbone upwards. Hold for 10 seconds and relax.

How many? 12–16

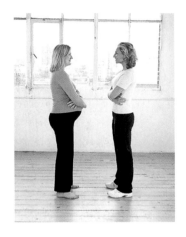

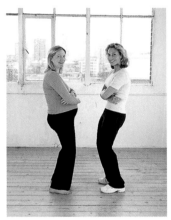

Standing Pelvic Tilt

What it does: Keeps the abdominal muscles in good condition.

What you do: Stand upright, maintaining good posture. Cross your arms over your belly drawing the abdominals together. Think about tightening your abdominal muscles as if to lift your baby up and in towards you. Hold for 10 seconds. This can be done standing, sitting or walking.

How many? 12–16

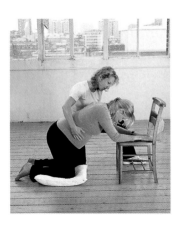

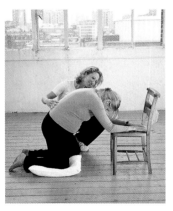

Abdominal Chair Tuck

What it does: Keeps the abdominal muscles in good condition.

What you do: Place a cushion under your knees and rest your body on your elbows on a chair in front of you. Contracting the abdominal muscles, arch the spine to the ceiling, visualizing your pelvis and breastbone being drawn close together.

How many? 12–16

Third Trimester

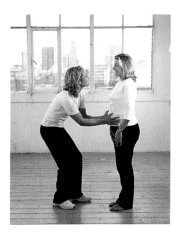
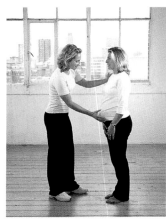

Standing Pelvic Tilt

What it does: Keeps the abdominal muscles in good condition.

What you do: Stand upright with good posture. Think about tightening your abdominal muscles as if to lift your baby up and in towards you. Hold for 10 seconds. This can be done standing, sitting or walking.

How many? 12–16

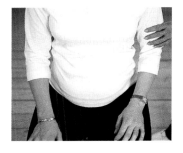
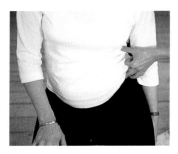

Seated Hip Hitch

What it does: Keeps the abdominal muscles in good condition.

What you do: Sit on a good supportive chair. Extend up through the spine. Focus on lifting one hip up towards the ribs, hold for 10 seconds and release. Repeat on the other side.

How many? 12–16 on each side

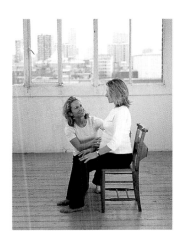
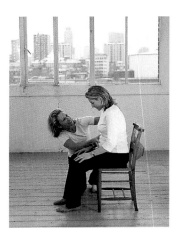

Seated Abdominal Curl

What it does: Keeps the abdominal muscles in good condition.

What you do: Sit with good posture with your hands resting on your thighs – or cross your arms over your belly and lightly clasp each side. Draw your baby in towards you, tilting your pelvis forwards and drawing your breastbone towards your pubic bone. Focus on tightening your abdominals. Hold for 10 seconds – make sure you don't hold your breath – and release.

How many? 12–16

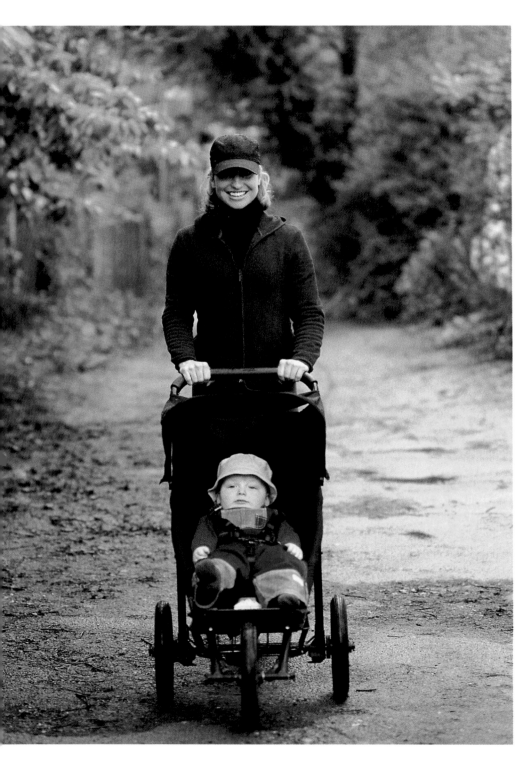

Post-natal

You may be keen to get back to your exercise routine and reclaim your body, but do have your post-natal check-up first. If you have had a Caesarean delivery, it is advisable to wait 8–10 weeks before exercising again. You can, however, start the following exercises before you have your check-up:

- **Pelvic tilts (see pages 147, 148, 149)**
- **Kegal exercise (see page 147)**
- **Static abdominal tightening exercises (see Rib-hip Connection, page 77)**

Once you have had the all-clear from your GP, remember to start out slowly. Your energy levels may be low through broken nights and breast-feeding. It is a good idea to use your baby's napping time as your physical investment time – which means thinking about resting as well as slotting in some of your toning exercises. Now is an excellent opportunity to focus on your posture and stability, which will have been affected by the change in your centre of gravity as your baby grew inside you. See pages 102 and 126 for these workouts. Try to do them 4 times a week, in addition to your abdominal work. While your baby is small, walking with your buggy can be a great way to introduce some cardio work. Slip on your trainers and your pedometer and build up those steps. See page 37 for walking tips.

Menopause

Proper nutrition and appropriate exercise play a fundamental part in health promotion and disease prevention for people of all ages. It is particularly effective when we experience the physiological and psychological changes associated with menopause. For many women menopause can be uncomfortable. But while no single exercise can prevent all the signs and symptoms of menopause, women can minimize the changes and positively influence their future health by exercising regularly.

What is menopause?

1. **Menopause represents the stage in a woman's life when her ovaries stop producing oestrogen and cease to release an egg each month.**
2. **It is most likely to occur between the ages of 41 and 59, the average age being 51.**
3. **Menopause is considered official when a woman has stopped menstruating for one year.**
4. **The physiological changes associated with menopause increase the risk of osteoporosis and heart disease.**

Signs and symptoms

Menopause symptoms occur as the body produces less and less oestrogen. Signs can start a year or more before the final period, and include changes in the menstrual cycle, vaginal dryness, excessive sweating, disrupted sleep, increased incidence of urinary tract infections, incontinence, dry skin, thinning hair and weight gain. This phase is known as the peri-menopause. Hot flushes are common due to the changing hormonal activity in the body. These physical changes can be very disturbing: women may experience erratic mood swings, feelings of losing control and depression.

Osteoporosis

Osteoporosis is often referred to as a 'paediatric disease with a geriatric face', as the actions we take in our earlier years can have a direct impact on our susceptibility to it in later life. However, when we hit menopause, the decline in oestrogen reduces our protection

Body laid bare

And now for the science bit…

Oestrogen helps to prevent bone loss, so a woman's bone density can significantly decrease during menopause, making her more vulnerable to osteoporosis and bone fracturing.

The body also produces higher amounts of the hormone insulin, which is responsible for stabilizing our blood glucose levels. This, coupled with the fact that the cells can become less receptive to glucose and less able to keep blood glucose levels constant, means that women can be at greater risk of diabetes and energy fluctuations. The body also changes the way it transports blood fats. Less favourable, low-density lipoproteins increase, and there is a rise in total plasma cholesterol levels. Both are associated with a higher risk of heart disease.

against potential bone loss. Studies indicate a 3–5% decrease in bone density for 5–7 years post-menopause. In addition you are at greater risk if you are petite, thin, inactive, Caucasian, a heavy smoker, have a history of low calcium intake or have entered menopause early.

The right exercise during menopause is a physical health investment which only you can make for yourself. Even if you never have exercised before. your body will benefit. Regular exercise during menopause will:

- **Reduce risk of heart disease.**
- **Help maintain bone density.**
- **Help maintain healthy body composition.**
- **Provide an important sense of control while your body is going through change.**
- **Potentially alleviate menopausal symptoms.**

Osteoporosis-specific Abdominal Exercises

If you already have osteoporosis you can still exercise, but you need to make certain adaptations to give you an effective exercise programme. Here are three abdominal exercises suitable for someone with osteoporosis in the vertebrae.

Body kit

Mat

The workout

Wall Roll-down (see page 100) x 4

Side Bend (see page 99) x 4, right and left

Shoulder Roll (see page 175) x 8

Side Leg Slide x 8, right and left

Single Bent Knee Lift x 8, right and left

Knee Lift with Leg Slide x 8, right and left

TOP TIP: If you are new to these exercises, start with 4 repetitions, building up to 8. Do not compromise your technique.

Basic Recommendations

* **20–60 minutes of cardiovascular exercise 3–5 times a week.**
* **Resistance training 2 days a week.**

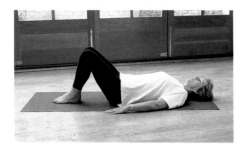

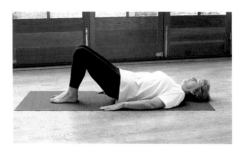

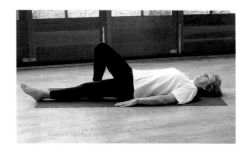

Single Leg Slide

What it does: Helps to tighten the abdominal area without placing strain on the spinal vertebrae.

What you do: Lie on your back with the knees bent, feet flat on the floor and arms at your sides. First perform a pelvic tilt. Exhale while sliding one leg forwards as far as possible, keeping the heel on the floor. Hold for 3 seconds. Maintaining the pelvic tilt, inhale and return to the starting position. Relax the pelvic tilt and repeat with the other leg.

How many? 8–12 on each leg

Top Tip: Make sure the waist stays on the floor. Shoes and socks can be removed to make it easier to slide the feet.

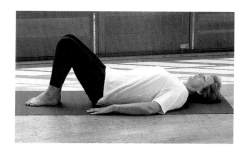 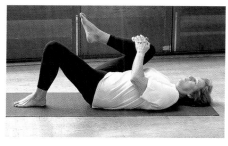

Single Bent Knee Lift

What you do: Lie on your back with the knees bent, feet flat on the floor and arms at your sides. Inhale and lift your leg 30cm/12in off the floor and bring the knee of that leg towards the chest. Exhale and return to the starting position. Repeat with other the leg.

Top Tips: Focus on pulling the abdominals up and in, as if drawing them under the ribs. The lower back should be flat on the floor. For a more advanced move, bring the thigh up to a 90° angle instead of all the way in to the chest.

How many? 8–12 on each leg

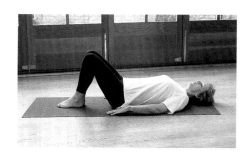 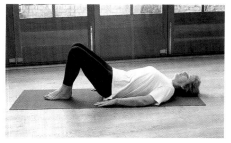

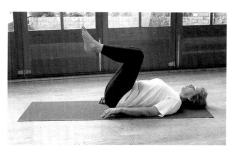 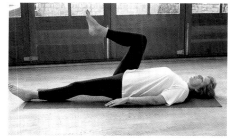

Knee Lift With Leg Slide

What it does: Helps to tighten the abdominal area without placing strain on the spinal vertebrae.

What you do: Lie on your back with the knees bent, feet flat on the floor and arms at your sides. Perform a pelvic tilt. Bring the knees in to the chest. Exhale and slowly slide one leg straight down along the floor back to the starting position. The heel should be in contact with the floor. Repeat on the other side.

Top Tip: Establish a neutral spine to prevent the lower back from arching.

How many? 8–12 on each leg

Case Study

Jane, a 45-year-old teacher, was diagnosed as having osteoporosis in her spine. Although she had never done any weight training, she was active, and walked 3.2km/2 miles every day and swam twice a week. She had suffered from lactose intolerance all her life, which had contributed to her low calcium intake.

Jane's Programme

As Jane already has osteoporosis in her spine, she needs to avoid:

- Forward flexion (bending forward from the hips)
- Twisting of the spine
- Jarring movements
- Any activity that could cause her to fall.

Lifestyle Recommendations

1. Continue with daily walking. Try to find routes that include inclines, declines and steps to increase impact forces through the legs without causing excessive jarring.
2. Introduce a simple step class at weekend.

Resistance Training

This should be undertaken on 2 days a week with a personal trainer or in a gym.

Jane practised an upper and lower body workout with resistance bands for 2 months. She then progressed to 2.25kg/5lb hand-held weights and ankle weights. For the first year Jane was advised not to increase the weight but rather to vary the exercises and the number of sets of exercises performed.

Jane's Sample Workout

Torso

Lat Pull-downs (see page 85), Seated Rows with Resistance Band (see page 85), Wall Push-ups (see page 180), Inclined Bench Press (see page 89).

Arms

Biceps Curls seated with weights, Lateral Raises with Resistance Band (see page 184), Triceps Dips (see page 194).

Legs

Sitting on chair and getting up without using hands.

Seated leg extension without weights, then add ankle weights (sit on a chair with good posture, knees over ankles, feet flat on the floor, lift one leg to straighten at the knee, and lower).

Standing leg curls with ankle weights (stand with good posture – you may wish to hold on to a wall or chair for balance with this exercise – and, keeping your knees together, bend the leg at the knee to bring the heel back towards your bottom, then lower).

Standing heel and toe raises (rise up on to your toes, lifting your heels).

Single Leg Presses, lying on your side or standing with chair for support (see page 83). Inner Thigh Leg Lifts, lying on your side (see page 83).

Back

Cobra with Arm Support (see page 86)

Abdominals

Specific abdominal work, as on pages 152–3.

Case Study

Mary is a 54-year-old divorced accountant. Her body weight is 74kg/11st 10lb. Mary used to go to the gym regularly until 2 years ago, but her hectic work schedule now requires her to travel abroad every 2 weeks, which has put an end to her gym workouts. She is on HRT and has gained weight – especially around her waist, upper back and backs of arms. She feels low, lethargic and flabby. She wants to lose excess weight around her middle and see some definition in her upper body, especially the troublesome backs of her arms.

Mary's Programme

Since osteoporosis is not a concern for Mary, she can do regular abdominal work and twisting in her programme. I also recommended some deep breathing and relaxation technique exercises at the end of each session to reduce her stress levels.

Lifestyle Recommendations

Mary needed to try to create some space for herself in her life. She has undergone a great deal of stress, both in her career and personally. She needed to address becoming generally more active, so she was set minimum of 4,000 steps a day on her pedometer. This could be incorporated into the periods of her day when she felt most under stress. I encouraged Mary to walk for 10 minutes first thing in the day and 10 minutes at lunchtime to try to achieve her walking targets. We developed the 10 minutes' walking target in the morning as Mary's planning time for her day ahead, and as she generally went out to lunch or bought herself a sandwich, which she ate at her desk, she was encouraged to walk for 20 minutes instead of the usual 10 before she opened her wallet to buy her lunch. This way Mary could justify her time away from her desk and easily slot in her walking targets.

Cardiovascular Programme

Mary was advised to achieve a 7,000 daily walking count 3 days a week. This could be slotted into her travelling schedule. On wet and rainy days, Mary can use a treadmill and stationary bike at about 5.6km/3.5 miles per hour for 20–30 minutes.

Mary's Sample Resistance Workout

Perform twice a week:

Back

One-arm rows 3.6kg/8lb	2 x 10
Back extensions	x 20

Legs

Swiss ball wall squats (hold bottom position for 5 seconds)	x 10
Outer and Inner Thigh Leg Lifts, lying on side (see page 83)	2 x 10

Arms

Triceps kick backs 2.25kg/5lb	2 x 10
Biceps curls 2.25kg/5lb	2 x 10
Lateral Raises (see page 184)	2 x 10
Alternating Frontal Raise with Resistance Band (see page 185)	2 x 10

Chest

Inclinded Bench Presses 3.6kg/8lb (see page 69)	2 x 10
Bench Presses 2.25kg/5lb (see page 89)	2 x 10
Wall Press-ups (see page 181)	x 16

Shoulders

Standing Shoulder Openings with Resistance Band (see page 186)	2 x 10

Abdominals

Abdominal body bar curls (see page 80)	x 16
Ball Offerings (see page 81)	x 16
Pelvic Tilts (see page 147)	x 16

High blood cholesterol

Many people have elevated blood cholesterol, which is a major risk factor in heart disease. Various therapies are available, including medication, dietary modification and exercise. Exercise has a very important part to play in reducing cholesterol levels, as it directly affects the blood lipid (blood fat) profile. However, it should be used to supplement drug therapy, if necessary, and diet modification. The benefits of exercise in controlling blood cholesterol come about with continued adherence to an exercise programme, so here is a sample programme:

Cholesterol-lowering Plan

Short-term goals:
- Initiate a specific walking programme – 3 times a week, 15 minutes each session.
- Add an additional exercise session each week, building up to 15 minutes, 6 times a week.
- Increase exercise time by 5 minutes each week.

Long-term goals:
- Achieve an exercise calorie burn greater than 1,000 calories per week.
- Include aerobic exercise activities that use the whole body, such as brisk walking, cycling or swimming. Exercise at a moderate intensity (40–70% of your maximum heart rate – see page 40) several days a week.
- You can achieve the desired energy burn by breaking your exercise sessions down into blocks or bouts.

High blood pressure

About 50 million people in the USA alone are thought to have high blood pressure (hypertension), and 1 in every 6 people in the UK. Hypertension puts you at greater risk of cardiovascular diseases, kidney failure and stroke. Individuals with the condition should take aerobic exercise 3–7 days per week for 20–60 minutes at 40–70% maximum oxygen uptake, or exercise at an RPE of 11–13 (see page 41).

Resistance exercise should be focused on more repetitions at lower resistance levels.

NB! ANYONE WITH A RESTING BLOOD PRESSURE OF 200/105 OR ABOVE SHOULD NOT PARTICIPATE!

Those who are overweight should also focus on effective weight loss. A 4.5kg/ 10lb decrease in your weight will create a 10mm Hg decrease in blood pressure.

Exercise for weight loss

Exercising to lose weight and achieve a healthy body fat level are among the main motivators that get us moving. However, exercise without dieting tends to have only a small effect on total body mass and body fat loss. The American College of Sports Medicine acknowledges that 'the most effective and successful studies in terms of weight loss have been those that combined diet and exercise' to optimize energy expenditure.

For weight management purposes, the most important issue is to burn as many calories as possible in each session, as well as accumulating energy expenditure through daily activity. Aim to achieve an energy expenditure of 250–300 calories per session as a minimum, 3 times a week. An energy expenditure of 200 calories per session may be effective if carried out at least 4 times each week. This expenditure is best achieved through aerobic activity. Supplementing your programme with resistance training will stimulate muscle mass and boost your metabolic rate.

Top Tip: Invest in a pedometer and aim to accumulate 10,000 steps each day. Studies have shown that this number of steps contributes to weight loss.

keeping motivated

By this stage you may have the exercise bug between your teeth, but what happens when your motivation starts to wane? Being prepared for lapses in your motivation is half the battle. Here are some tips to keep you going when the going gets tough.

Be brutally honest!

Make a list of reasons why you want to shed the weight, get fitter and improve your body shape. Think hard, dig deep and list absolute truths. Being healthier is a good reason but it might not be the real issue for you. You may find it difficult to commit to paper something like 'I find it difficult having sex because I feel uncomfortable about my body', but if this is the real reason, then write it down!

Log your workouts

Keeping a training journal can be a great way to quantify your progress. It is so much better than guesswork, and can keep you on schedule for your training goal (see page 158 for a sample journal).

If you cross-train, it is a good idea to divide your training journal into sections: one for cardio/aerobic exercise and one for strength/resistance activity – and maybe one for mind-body workouts.

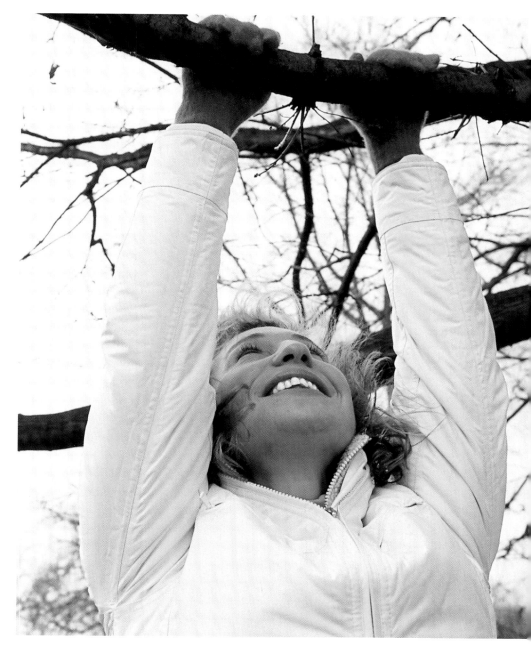

Sample training journal

Cardio/aerobic activity

Date	Exercise	Distance	Time	Notes
May 11	Treadmill	4 km	29 mins	This was a slower time than normal – started the workout a little dehydrated – must remember to drink more during the day next week. Get time back down to 25 minutes.
May 15	Spinning class	Varied	45 mins	
May 16	Workout video	Cardio calorie burn	20 mins	Short on time today, off travelling to Europe with business, so just squeezed in this workout before I left for work.

Strength/resistance activity

Date	Exercise	Repetitions	Sets	Weight Used	Notes
May 10	Bench press	6	1	64kg/140lb	
	Dumbbell press	12	1	10kg/22lb	
	Chest flyes	12	1	10kg/22lb	
May 15	Leg press	12	1	73kg/160lb	This is first time I have done a leg session after my spinning class. Legs definitely felt it.
	Leg curl	12	1	30kg/66lb	

Mind-body activity

Date	Exercise	Class	Notes
May 17	Yoga	Hatha Yoga beginners, Week 1	Started 6-week course on advice from personal trainer. This should definitely make me more disciplined about my stretching programme!

Exercise supporter or saboteur?

It is always a good idea to find yourself a training buddy. You can keep each other motivated, and on track. But choose your partner carefully. Make sure they are going to be there to encourage you and not to tempt you to grab a cappuccino or a glass of wine when their motivation starts to slack. If you have a tendency to drop off your exercise, discipline yourselves to see and chat to each other only when you are doing your workouts. Avoid chatting on the phone between workouts. This will provide an additional incentive to see that person each workout and keep them up-to-date with what is going on in your life.

Set realistic goals

As with any business, if you want to achieve something you have to set goals. These need to be realistic and quantifiable. Announcing 'I'm going to drop 20lb in 3 weeks' is neither realistic nor healthily achievable. Instead try this: 'I have my weekend away with my friends in 3 weeks, and I'd really like to feel I have more energy and fit into my clothes a little better. So, this week I will:

- Do the Seated Sun Salutation workout (see page 195) 4 times before I go to work.
- Accumulate 6,000 steps each day on my pedometer.
- Complete the Best Body Bits abdominal workout (page 79) times.

Reward yourself

Everyone likes to get a present, so why not give yourself a gift on completion of your goals? Make it a treat that complements your health improvements – maybe a body wrap from your beauty therapist, a new set of workout kit, or a new bike to enjoy with the family. Avoid treats that could conflict with your health improvements – while a meal with your friends may be great fun, if you are new to exercise and know your resistance to temptation is weak, you may be inclined to over-indulge and end up feeling guilty the following day.

Make it a date

If you don't plan your exercise, all too often it is the exercise that gets left off the 'To Do' list. Make an appointment with yourself and put it in your diary. This may sound boring, but your physical activity is an investment in yourself that only you can make.

Change your attitude!

Try to develop an appreciation that exercise is not just about burning calories but has many other benefits that you may not at first appreciate. It increases your alertness, lessens stress and energizes you. So you feel like skipping a workout? Stop! And remember ALL the good exercise does for you!

Suit yourself!

If you are off to the gym to work out, go at the best time for you. Maybe you like it when the gym is buzzing – perhaps this motivates you more – or maybe you find the busiest times a little intimidating. Speak to your gym instructors and, if you have some flexibility in your schedule, select a time that creates the best environment for you to achieve your fitness and health goals.

Be regular!

There must be something you do every day – maybe it's buying your coffee on the way to work, your train tickets at the station, a sandwich at lunch, or perhaps posting a letter. Whatever it is, resolve to move your body for 10 minutes before you do it. Use this time to think about the day ahead – plan your shopping list or prepare a presentation. Your exercise activity time need never be wasted time.

Become a Weekend Warrior

If you struggle to find time to exercise during the week, look to your weekends as an opportunity to enjoy your physical activity pursuits. If you have battled with your weight time and time again, and this is your main focus for keeping fit – then ditch that goal and find yourself an event to work towards. It could be a 5km/3.1 mile fun run, a sponsored walk or a marathon. Select something that is going to challenge you physically. As you work towards achieving your goal, you will experience other benefits such as weight loss and increased self-esteem – even though this was not your primary goal. One of the main reasons why working towards an event is so effective is that you cannot move the goalposts. You can let yourself off when you don't achieve your weight loss target at the end of the month, even move it to next month, but with an event you do not have that escape route. You can try ringing up the race organizers, explaining your training has not gone too well and asking if they can put the event back a month, but it is unlikely to help!

Recruit a personal trainer

You may think having a personal trainer is a luxury only for the rich and famous, but even if you can't afford a full-time trainer, recruiting the services of a PT when you know you habitually experience a decrease in your motivation or just plain stop exercising can get you over those hurdles. Maybe it is the February blues, when your new motivation has worn off, or perhaps you are having problems seeing that extra definition in your arms when you want to look amazing for a wedding coming up. Instead of giving up, use the help at hand to get you over those problem times. A good PT will be able to guide you and educate you to feel the benefits of their expertise well after the training sessions have finished.

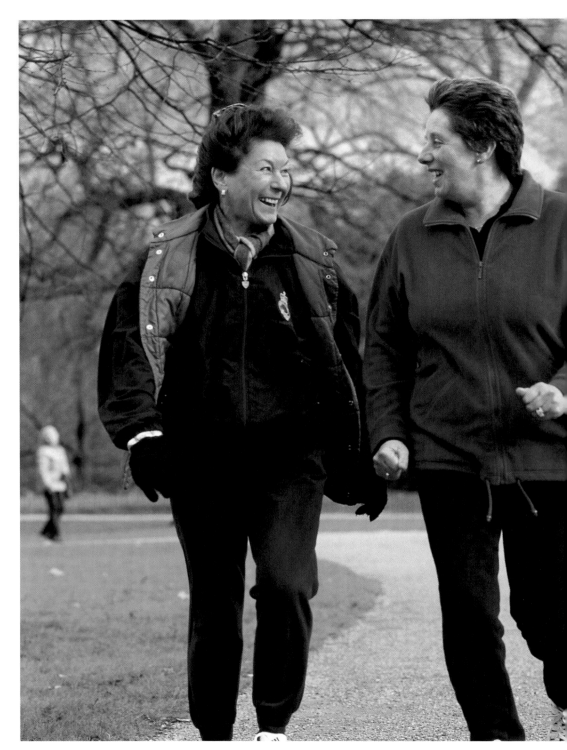

exercise and health through the decades

Let's face it – at one time or another we have all wanted to stop the hands of time. In fact 3 out of every 5 of us want to live to 100, according to a recent survey. So far science, despite the enormous advances made over the past century, has not been able to turn back the clock. However, much of what we consider to be the effects of ageing may well result from a lifelong accumulation of inadequate nutrition and activity. And there is no doubt that the quality and quantity of exercise that we have taken throughout our lives does, quite literally, shape our bodies.

But what type of exercise should we take?

Aerobic exercise has been shown to improve cardiovascular health, but does not seem to influence muscle mass or muscle strength. Resistance training, on the other hand, has a potent effect in both these areas, and also appears to have a positive impact on our bone density and dynamic balance. Studies have demonstrated that aerobic activity and strengthening exercises can reduce depressive symptoms and sleep problems in older adults. Improving mood and sleep is essential to the quality of life.

As we get older, the demands we place on our bodies, and what we expect from them, alters. This is a result of physiological changes as well as self-neglect. Studies have shown that from the age of 25 our aerobic capacity decreases by 1–2% every year. Since many of us are now living well into our 80s and beyond, the loss of aerobic capacity for many individuals means that the normal daily activities – such as getting out of bed – will require significant effort to accomplish. As this continues there develops a very fragile threshold between dependency and self-sufficiency. But it's not just in the golden years that lack of physical care for our bodies can erode the quality of our lives. Not many people realize that, starting in their mid-30s, women lose 140–170g/5–6oz of muscle each year and gain as much, if not more, fat mass. Compounding the issue is the fact that at progressive life stages our motivation towards our physical health alters, and faces different lifestyle constraints.

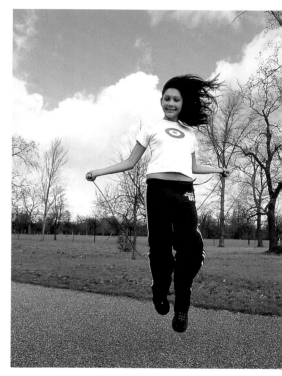

Following is a quick reference guide for putting together an action plan to age-proof our bodies through the decades. You shouldn't wait till after 40 to begin looking after your body, but if you have, that's okay – remember that every little thing you do will make a difference. No matter how old or young you are, your body can still benefit from exercise.

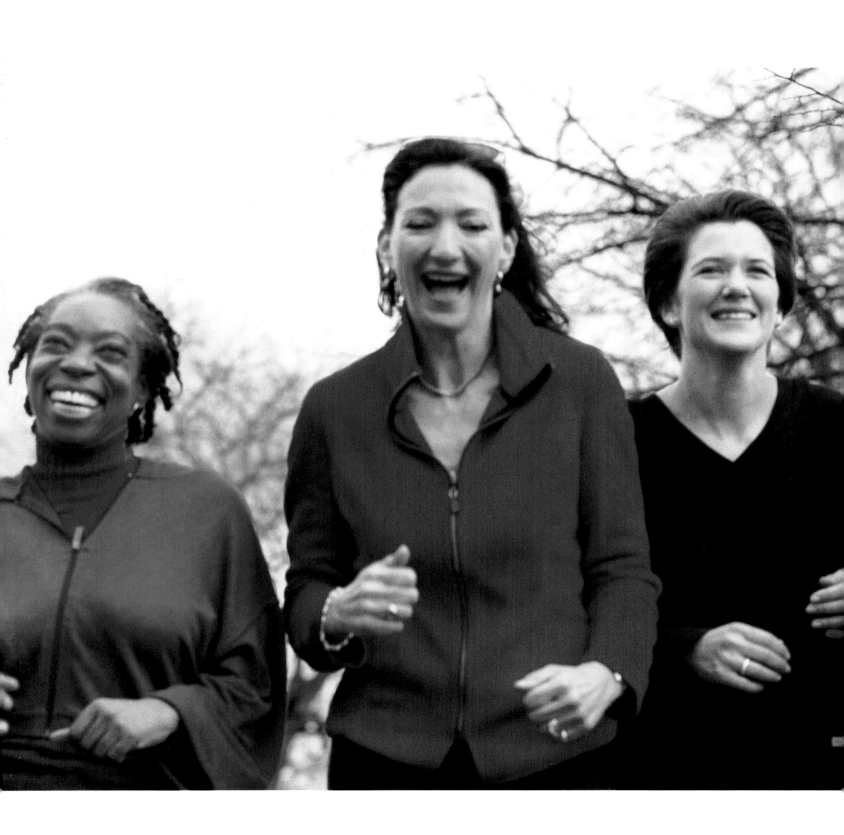

In your 20s:

STOP... depriving yourself of water and sleep.

The niggling health problems that can make a misery of your 20s – such as headaches, eczema, depression, irritable bowel syndrome, bad skin and pre-menstrual syndrome (PMS) – often improve dramatically when you cut down on alcohol and junk food and increase your intake of water and sleep.

Water is a medium for the removal of all our waste products and the toxins that we put into our body (see page 219). Aim to drink at least 2 litres/3½ pints a day. Sleep generates greater creativity and emotional balance, and improves short-term memory and problem-solving capabilities. Studies have also found that social drinkers who cut down on alcohol find themselves less anxious and depressed, and experience fewer mood swings.

START... getting into the exercise habit.

It may be a little while since you were playing sport at school, but don't let the absence of physical exercise become the norm. Get into the habit of taking regular structured exercise 2–3 times a week. Focus on cardiovascular activity to build up the stamina of your heart and lungs and to maintain your aerobic capacity. Experiment with mind-body exercise such as yoga to provide a balance in a perhaps frantic social life and boost body awareness.

THINK ABOUT... the price of convenience.

Smoking (passive or active), convenience food and alcohol mean 20-somethings often end up with an antioxidant deficit. Antioxidants have been linked to the prevention of numerous conditions from heart disease and cancer to cataracts and arthritis. To rebalance, eat more fruit, vegetables and grains of various kinds. Consider taking an antioxidant supplement (vitamins A, C and E, and minerals selenium, copper and zinc). Evening primrose oil can reduce pre-menstrual water retention and breast tenderness (though the effects may take a few months to kick in) and vitamin B complex and magnesium may help with pre-menstrual problems that are more emotional than physical.

REMEMBER...

Women should go for regular cervical smears, and also a chlamydia test. Studies that 1 in 20 sexually active women may have chlamydia.

In your 30s:

STOP... smoking.

If asthma, chest infections, bronchitis and various respiratory diseases haven't made you pack it in already, stop now! The risk of lung cancer increases exponentially if you have smoked for more than 20 years. As soon as you stop, your lungs start recovering.

START... to introduce some resistance exercise to your regular aerobic programme.

There are hundreds of reasons to exercise. Here are 5 to motivate you in your 30s.

1. Muscle mass starts to decline in your 20s, so you could be heading for an increase in your fat mass. In you are not doing weight bearing, by age 39 you could potentially have lost 1.8kg/4lb of muscle mass and replaced it with body fat.
2. Fitter people have better circulation, which means a higher sex drive – important for women, who reach their sexual peak in their 30s.
3. Exercise is one of the most effective ways to control stress – whether you are a wife, mother or career-woman, the stresses of everyday life can be at their height right now.
4. The heart muscle needs exercise to remain strong. Staying fit lowers the risk of heart disease, diabetes and strokes, and raises oxygen levels in the body, keeping the brain alert.
5. Developing core strength through mind-body exercise such as Pilates will reduce your risk of back pain and help to maintain a lean, flat torso.

THINK ABOUT... stress levels.

Everyone needs space and solitude to relax. There are very few health problems – physical or mental – which are not related to stress. Find your stress outlet, whether it's yoga, swimming, walking or pottering about in the garden. Vitamin B complex helps the functioning of the brain and nervous system. St John's wort can alleviate mild to moderate bouts of depression.

REMEMBER...
Check moles for changes in colour and shape.

In your 40s:
STOP... middle-age spread.
Insomnia, impotence, osteoporosis and diabetes are all linked to weight gain and inactivity. Lack of flexibility is one of the strongest indicators of ageing – so start a stretching programme and make sure you achieve a minimum of 30 minutes' daily physical activity. This activity needs to become the foundation of your future health as moderate exercise has been shown to have the greatest impact on reducing blood pressure, insensitivity to glucose – which is an early indication of late-onset diabetes – and also on positively changing our blood lipid profile.

START... eating more fruit and fibre.
30–50% of cancers are thought to be preventable if people adhered to a healthier diet. Bowel cancer, for example, is directly related to intake of fibre, fat and water. Heart disease is also strongly linked to diet: oily fish (fresh mackerel, tuna, salmon and tinned sardines) protect against heart disease by increasing beneficial high-density lipoproteins.

THINK ABOUT... fish oil and vitamin E supplements.
Through their effect on the blood, fish oils help lower our blood cholesterol levels, improve circulation and ease arthritis. Vitamin E has also been linked with a reduced risk of prostate cancer and heart disease.

REMEMBER...
Ask your doctor to check your blood pressure and perhaps arrange a bone density scan.

In your 50s:
STOP... standing on your bathroom scales!
Instead monitor your body composition and specifically your body fat. You can use body fat monitoring devices in your home or at the gym. Muscle weighs more than fat, and while your weight may be similar to your weight in your 30s, your percentage body fat may have increased, placing you at greater risk of heart disease, diabetes and some cancers.

START... drinking 8 glasses of water a day.
By 50 our thirst mechanism can be suppressed, creating a situation where our body is chronically dehydrated. Cross-sectional studies are now indicating that even drinking 6 glasses of water a day instead of 8 can leave us chronically dehydrated. This has been linked to gall stones, kidney stones and bowel and prostate cancer.

THINK ABOUT... taking up t'ai chi.
Studies have shown that this discipline is one of the best ways to stimulate brain-eye co-ordination and improve body awareness. Studies on stroke victims found a significant improvement in recovery rates with regular t'ai chi.

REMEMBER... to have a regular health test.
Everyone should ask their doctor for a bowel cancer test, and women should have a mammogram every 3 years for the rest of their life. Those with a family history of breast or ovarian cancer may also want to be screened for ovarian cancer.

In your 60s:
STOP... doing high-impact workouts, and change your routine with more moderate and longer-duration exercise.
The risk of arthritis is greater in this age group, and more moderate, low-impact activity such as walking, swimming and t'ai chi will not place undue stress on the legs.

START... Mental exercises.
Never done the crossword at the back of the newspaper? Now is the time to start.

THINK ABOUT... having an annual 'flu jab, because 'flu can be far more dangerous when you are in your 60s.

REMEMBER...

To play with your grandchildren – and if you don't have grandchildren of your own, make a concerted effort to be amongst younger people. It will keep you both physically and mentally on the ball!

In your 70s:

START... to use your chronobiological rhythm!

Everyone has chronobiological peaks and troughs, and these relate to the physiological, psychological and cognitive functioning of our body. Take physical exercise when your body is on a chronobiological down time and it will be harder to keep going and sustain motivation.

STOP... thinking this is it!

In a study of the 'super young', 3,500 people who seemed exceptionally young for their age found that one of the biggest contributing factors in retaining youthfulness was the continual development of friendships and interests.

THINK ABOUT... measuring your blood pressure regularly, either through your GP or with a home device.

High blood pressure can alert you to the danger of heart disease or strokes.

REMEMBER...

To have a bone scan to measure the density of your bones. In your 70s you run a higher risk of fractures from falls.

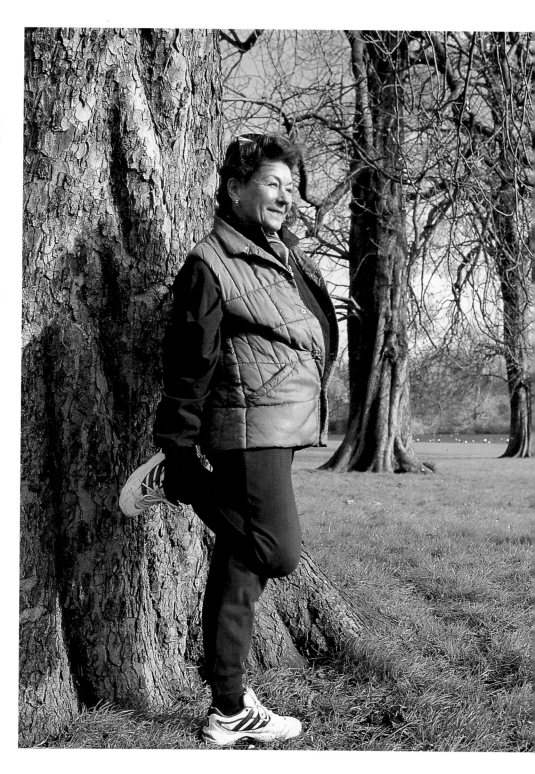

lifestyle challenges

Navigating your day

Now that most of us are leading life on the technology superhighway, the world of work can be frantic and stressful, and leave us very little time for ourselves – let alone an opportunity to take some structured exercise. Sometimes all we can do is hang on and hope we don't get tossed out along the way. The result? Energy-sapping, nerve-racking worry elevates our stress hormone (cortisol) levels. Research indicates that chronic exposure to elevated cortisol contributes to increased levels of fat deposition (specifically around our midriffs), which in turn is said to contribute to a 3–5-fold increase in the risk of certain diseases.

Day-in, day-out stress affects our posture and produces lethargy and body pain. From morning to evening our body's nervous system hits peaks and troughs as we cope with a barrage of demands: deadlines, traffic jams, high-pressure meetings, the boss's moods and constant interruptions. Even when the ride is exhilarating, our nervous system still takes a battering. The human body was not designed for life on a roller-coaster. It is blasted with a constant bombardment of coffee, sugar, fast foods and snacks, and our inactive and sedentary lifestyle chained to a desk or with a telephone clamped to our ear compounds the problem. Instead of establishing a pleasant plateau of focus and energy in our life, we can find ourselves between frantic activity and sluggishness, as we experience adrenaline rushes, caffeine highs and blood glucose insulin rebounds.

But it does not have to be like this. If you are looking to even out the ride a bit, moving your body and making small changes to what you are eating and drinking can be hugely beneficial. Physical activity has been shown to be the best way to dissipate stress hormones. So here are some tips to help you become more stress-resilient and better prepared to cope with your daily work demands.

Even if your day doesn't revolve around an office and instead you have to cope with being at home with the kids, juggle a part-time job with your family commitments, or just lead a demanding social life, you can use the navigation path alongside as a guide to getting just a bit more activity into your day. Although not all the tips may be relevant, you can easily tailor them to fit your circumstances. Once they have become habits you will be more willing to experiment with others:

 06.00: Arghh – the alarm goes off. This may not be your normal waking hour, but whatever time you get up, experiment with rising a little earlier and don't turn off your alarm. If you can't bring yourself to spring out of bed at the first alarm, place the clock so you have to S-t-r-e-t-c-h to turn it off. Don't stop there. Keep stretching, stretch through your fingers and all the way down to your toes while still lying in your bed. Look at any animal and you will see it always stretches itself as it wakes up. Movement stimulates the waking part of the brain so you will find it easier to escape the gravitational pull of the pillow!

 06.15: Boil some water and complete the mobility or posture exercises (see pages 99–104) as you wait for it to boil. Make yourself a Wake-up Lemon Drink. **If you are short of time, just do 3 or 4 Seated Sun Salutations (see page 195)– they will increase the blood flow through the body, give you more energy and gradually raise your body temperature, which will have**

fallen during the night. Increasing the body temperature helps your body's metabolism and enzyme activity.

 07.00: Skip the caffeine and substitute a glass of freshly squeezed, diluted orange juice or grapefruit juice. Bypass the sugary cereals, which create a fast sugar rush and then bring you crashing down, and opt instead for a slow-releasing breakfast option such as porridge oats with berries, a breakfast smoothie or a slice of toast with a boiled egg (see Chapter 6 for more ideas). No time to eat now? Then grab a flask and do a breakfast on-the-go smoothie.

 08.00: Turn your commuting time into quiet time. If you drive, leave the radio off. If you commute, scan the papers selectively, check out the news-in-brief sections and then take a few moments to become aware of your breath and practise your 2:1 Breathing**. You'll find you come into the office more refreshed and less frazzled, having had a little time to be still.**

 09.00: Resolve to walk briskly for at least 10 minutes before you sit down at your desk. As the pace picks up in the office, you will be pleased you have kick-started your body. In the next hour drink a glass of water, and eat your breakfast if you have brought it with you.

 10.00: Quick posture check. Focus on how your body is positioned – it really won't take long. Check your feet are flat on the floor and you are extending through your spine, and consciously pull in your abdominal muscles to help keep the extension right up through your spine. Try to get up and move your body every 60 minutes – it will help stimulate blood flow to the brain and dissipate cortisol levels.

 11.00: As your colleagues reach for that mid-morning caffeine and sugar fix, try to opt for a piece of fruit instead, although you may not be wanting it if you have had a nutritious breakfast. Drink some fruit juice as well as water, or try real ginseng tea or coffee substitutes, such as chicory.

 12.00: Do some neck stretches and Upper Spine Rotation (see page 176). This will relieve tension in your upper body and reduce the compression through your lumbar vertebrae. If you have been working at a computer, try the Eyestrain Buster **(see page 168) to energize your eye–brain communication.**

 13.00: Try to avoid working through your lunch break. Even if you have a deadline to hit, don't skip your lunch. You need to eat something to replenish vital blood glucose – essential to help you concentrate – and a quick walk will help reduce your cortisol levels. So when you go out, make sure you walk for at

Wake-up Lemon Drink

Here's a drink that will wake up your excretory system. Boil a cup of water and mix it with the juice of a freshly squeezed lemon. Add a pinch of salt and, when the mixture is cool enough to drink, stir in up to a teaspoon of honey. The lemon juice cleanses the kidneys as well as the bowels, the salt will draw waste material from the bloodstream, and the honey soothes and tones the intestinal tract.

2:1 Breathing

This breathing pattern relaxes the body by subtly coaxing the parasympathetic nervous system (which controls the automatic functions such as the beating of the heart and the digestion) into a state of relaxation.

Gently slow down the rate of exhalation until you are exhaling twice as long as you are inhaling. You can achieve longer exhalations by contracting the abdomen slightly. Don't try to fill or empty the lungs completely – it may help to count to 6 on the exhalation and 3 on the inhalation, or 4 on the exhalation and 2 on the inhalation (or any 2:1 ratio you find comfortable). Focus on the smoothness and evenness of your breath, gradually eliminating all jerks and pauses.

Eyestrain Buster

This takes about 2 minutes and is great for relieving strained, tired eyes. Open your hands and gently slide the undersides of the thumbs across the upper rim of the eye sockets towards the temples. Then massage the lower rim of the eye sockets with your index fingers. Begin at the corners of your eyes and work towards the temples. Repeat twice more.

Now move your eyes slowly from side to side 3 times, slowly up and down 3 times, and finally in complete circles. Relax by closing your eyes so gently the eyelids barely touch.

Sleep Exercise

This great little technique will not only get you off to sleep but also help you sleep more peacefully. It uses an effortless 2:1 breath. Pay close attention to your breathing. There should not be any pauses, jerks or shakiness. Eliminate even the pause between the inhalation and exhalation.

Get into bed and take: 8 breaths
lying on your back;
16 breaths lying on your right side;
32 breaths lying on your left side.

Very few people complete this exercise. Sweet dreams!

least 10 minutes before you buy your lunch. Lunch can sap your energy, so make sure you choose wisely. Select a meal that combines several proteins, as this will stimulate the brain transmitter dopamine that makes us feel more alert, as well as some starch, which fuels our muscles' glycogen levels. Avoid too heavy a food intake, as this will drain your energy levels and leave you craving a sugar and caffeine fix to kick-start your afternoon.

 14.00: You're back at your desk, ready and feeling refreshed. Make sure that you drink a glass of water in the next hour. Reassess your posture and ensure that your shoulder blades are down and there is a good distance between your ears and your shoulders. Check your breathing, and make sure you are allowing the air to enter all the way into the body down to the diaphragm and not just to the chest. Chest breathing automatically triggers the nervous system.

 15.00: Starting to slump? Complete whatever you are in the middle of, then get up and move your body – even if that only means climbing a set of stairs or walking to the post box. You will return to your desk feeling more positive and able to continue with your 'To Do' list with renewed vigour. Can't get away from your desk? Then lower your chest to your thighs, link your arms under them, hold on at the elbows or forearms and pull up through the upper back. This relieves tension in the upper back and shoulder area.

 16.00: The classic vending-machine hour! Resist the urge for that sugar fix, but do allow yourself to eat a strategic snack if you feel hungry. Opt for something that will hydrate you, and that contains a little protein and natural sugar. Try a ginseng tea and a bio yoghurt, or a fruit smoothie. This will recharge your batteries and help curb your body's hunger pangs later.

 17.00–18.30: Your journey home can be a really challenging battle with those hunger pangs. As you walk out of the office, focus on your posture: make sure you extend up through your spine – visualize yourself as tall as possible. If you really can't resist the quick-fix snack urge resign yourself to walking briskly for 10 minutes before you buy anything. And make sure it is always a bottle of water first!

 19.00: This is your time to get a little hot and sweaty in your structured exercise (see pages 33–7 for ideas). If you tend to overeat at night, and especially if you have had a stressful day, focus on increasing the intensity of your workout efforts, even if this means reducing the length of your exercise session. Thirty minutes is all you need. Studies have shown that exercising at a higher intensity will actually suppress your appetite and decrease your levels of cortisol. In addition, current evidence suggests that exercising at varying intensities is far more beneficial in terms of weight loss than always working at a slow pace for a longer time.

 20.00: Your evening meal should include fresh vegetables, fruit, some grains and good-quality protein such as fish, lean meat and pulses. Try to have a range of different colours on your plate: this will boost your antioxidant intake as well as providing a richer variety of nutrients. Whatever you choose, try to keep it light, especially if you eat late. A heavy meal before bed will interfere with your sleep and you will feel sluggish when you need to wake up.

 21–22.00: Try to unwind with a relaxing and enjoyable activity. If you have a family, play a game or team up to prepare tomorrow's lunch or breakfast.

 23.00: How you go to sleep has everything to do with how you wake up. If you experience difficulty sleeping, try the Meditation **or** Systematic Relaxation **before getting into bed. Once in bed, try the** Sleep Exercise**.**

Meditation

The practice of meditation gently frees us from the worries and mental entanglements that gnaw away at our body as we respond to the needs of the moment. It does not have to be time-consuming. Even a few moments in the morning and 5 minutes in the evening before bed will calm the nervous system and soothe the mind. Find a quiet, private place. Sit on the floor with a cushion under you or in a firm chair, with your head and back straight and your eyes closed. Allow all your muscles to relax except those that are supporting your head, neck and back.

When your body is relaxed, bring your awareness to your breath. Let it come primarily from the diaphragm, leaving your chest and shoulders motionless. Experience your breathing in an open and accepting way. As thoughts come let them pass without reacting to them and continue to be aware of your breath. Gently repeat the words 'I am perfectly still' in your mind (see also page 98).

Systematic Relaxation

This is a great way to clear your mind of tension. It reduces stress while resting the mind and body. With constant practice you can learn to relax in the space of a few breaths. Lie on your back with a small pillow under your head, your palms up and your feet slightly spread. Allow the floor to support you and turn your attention to your breath for a few moments. Then mentally scan the body from head to toe and back again, pausing briefly to become aware of each area. Aim to release any tension you notice. Begin with the top of the head, then move to the forehead, face, jaws and ears. Continue to the throat, shoulders, upper arms, palms, fingers and fingertips. Return along the joints of the wrist, elbows and shoulders. Relax the spine, abdomen and pelvis, the buttocks, thighs, calves, shins, feet, toes and toe tips. Exhale and inhale 4 times as though your whole body is exhaling and inhaling. Exhale all your worries and anxieties. Inhale vital energy, tranquillity and peace.

Become aware of the joints of the toes, the ankles, knees and hips. Relax the vertebrae from the coccyx to the base of the neck. Relax the head and the top of the head. Exhale from the head to the tips of the toes and inhale from the toe tips back to the top of the head. Repeat this 3 times. Be aware of the calm flow of the breath. Make a gentle effort to guide your breath so that it remains smooth and deep without jerks or pauses. Gently open your eyes. Stretch and notice how you feel. Try to maintain this feeling of calmness.

Lack of sleep

After exercise, sleep is usually the next item to be shoved off the 'To Do' list. One of the worst things you can do to your body is to neglect your pillow time. Rest is crucial if your body is to benefit from the physiological responses that are occurring as your fitness improves. Without proper rest, you will not have the energy to expend on exercise. A regular bedtime and a consistent time of rising will do wonders for your sleep.

The quality of your sleep can have an impact your hormone levels. The deep REM (rapid eye movement) sleep boosts the immune system, while lack of it diminishes production of the human growth hormone (hGH), which naturally diminishes in women as they approach menopause. As hGH levels drop, energy plummets because lean muscle tissue slowly decreases. Lower levels of hGH therefore lead to a lowered metabolic rate as metabolically active tissue decreases. If you have problems sleeping, practise the Sleeping Exercise on page 168.

Quiet Eyes

Have you ever found yourself waking in the middle of the night and noticed that when you try to drop back off to sleep your mind is already racing? When the mind races, your eyes will also be flickering, reflecting the activity of your brain. If you can still your eyes, you will find you will be able to still the mind. Practise the Quiet Eyes exercise to help you quiet your brain.

Lie in a comfortable, relaxing space face-up, eyes shut. Keeping your eyes shut, cast them down towards your navel, and try to focus your attention on that one spot. Take 5 deep breaths as you keep your eyes drawn towards that spot. Notice that as your mind starts to wander so does your eye-line. Try to keep the eyes directed towards the navel again and focus on letting them soften and fall away from your eyelids. All the time be aware of your breath. You may find it helps to practise Quiet Eyes as you listen to the Relaxation Meditation (see page 98).

Stress

Stress is now a common factor in everyday life. Chronic long-term stress can cause weight gain as a consequence of residual levels of the stress hormone cortisol in the bloodstream. Cortisol leads to an accelerated breakdown of lean muscle tissue and an enhanced deposition of body fat, especially in the trunk, neck and face. While stress can initially cause weight loss, weight gain can occur several months after the initial cause.

Stress also disturbs the balance of a number of key body functions, as it can affect the thyroid gland, sex hormones and pancreatic hormones. It triggers eating behaviours that cause weight gain, as sufferers experience cravings for sugar and salty food.

The most effective way to minimize cortisol levels in the blood is with regular physical activity and stress-relieving techniques such as meditation and mind-body exercises (see the Meditation on page 98, the yoga workouts on page 113 and the yoga postures below). Also invest in a pedometer to ensure you are accumulating your daily physical activity. This will help if the very fact that you cannot make your structured exercise session is itself causing you anxiety.

One-hit wonders

Remember to exhale into postures and inhale as you come out of them. The duration of the postures listed below should be lengthened as the body grows stronger and the healing aspects of the pose become apparent.

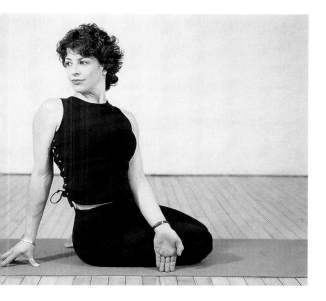

Mermaid (Bharadvajasana)

What it does: Eases lower back pain. Increases flexibility in the lower back and hip area. Can bring relief to stiffness and pain in the lumbar spine. Has overall benefits for the spine as well as helping to release the shoulders and discomfort in the neck.

What you do: Sit in Dandasana (see page 121), with palms flat on the floor behind your buttocks and all fingers pointing forwards. Bend your knees and move your shins to the left, ensuring that both knees and thighs point forwards.

Draw the shins closer to you with your left hand, so that both feet are in line with the left hip. The arch of the right foot will support the front of your left ankle.

The buttocks remain on the floor and help in lengthening and lifting the spine.

With your left hand placed on your right knee, take the right hand round behind you with the fingers pointing away from the body. The left shoulder blade will be tucked in and the right one will move back. Pressing downwards into the right shin will help to create further rotation to the right. The aim is to bring the left side of your body in line with your right thigh. Be careful that you don't force your neck and that you turn your head without discomfort.

Repeat to the left.

How long? Hold for 8–10 breaths.

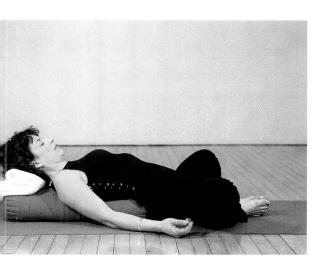

Reclining Butterfly (Supta Baddaknonasana)

What it does: Relieves pre-menstrual tension. Improves circulation to and function of the reproductive organs. Assists in regulating blood pressure. Helps to reduce anxiety and stress.

What you do: It is best to lie along a bolster, to help support the lower back and also release the shoulders and upper back. As the posture is practised for its remedial benefits, it is also helpful to have support under the knees and under the head. If you have nothing else, a blanket can be folded and evenly pleated to support the length of the spine and neck. Wooden blocks or telephone directories can placed under both knees

and a folded towel will do for under the head.

With the bolster or blanket behind you and against your buttocks and the folded towel at its end, under your head, bend the knees and bring the soles of the feet in towards you, allowing the knees to drop apart.

Take the elbows on to the floor behind you, and gently lower yourself down on to the bolster, ensuring that the head is comfortably supported. Feel the spine aligned with the bolster and the knees and neck able to relax. Allow your arms to rest away from your body, with the palms facing the ceiling. Relax and enjoy the benefits of the pose with your eyes closed. Turn and rest on your side to come out of the posture.

How long? Hold for 20 breaths.

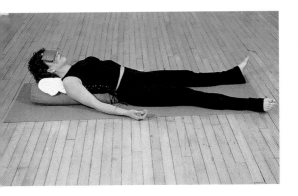

Corpse (Savasana)

What it does: Therapeutic for headaches, migraines, stress-related anxiety and insomnia. The simple nature of this posture helps to focus the mind, drawing it into a state of deep relaxation that is highly restorative and healing. It increases the function of the immune system.

What you do: Use a bolster or pleated blanket under the spine and supporting the neck to raise the chest and diaphragm and clear the mind. Use a lavender bag over your eyes to soothe the pain, ensure lights are dimmed and that you are warm and unlikely to be disturbed.

Lie down with the bolster positioned against your buttocks and with your head resting on a folded towel or blanket. Let your legs stretch out away from you about hip-width apart. Let the feet fall away from each other and the thighs soften and relax. Lift and separate the buttocks to release the lower back further. Be aware of the sound and movement of your breath, as you allow your arms to extend away from your body with your palms facing the ceiling.

Take a long and slow breath in and exhale with a long sigh, relaxing the throat as you do so. Let the shoulders draw down to lengthen the neck and allow your tongue to rest back away from the teeth on your palate. With lips together and teeth apart, relax deep into the hinges of your jaw and soften all the muscles in your cheeks and under your eyes. Allow the eyes to look inwards and downwards and focus your attention on stillness from within. Experience a true sense of union between the mind and the body, shared by the breath. Stay in the pose for 10 minutes or more.

Turn on to your right side when you have stretched in the pose and rest there for at least 20 breaths.
How long? Hold for 20 breaths.

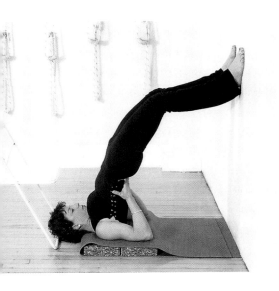

Supported Plough (Supported Halasana)

What it does: Helps combat insomnia. Helps symptoms of fatigue and exhaustion and promotes deep dreamless sleep. Helps to soothe and clear discomfort from a sore throat, blocked nose or chest infection. Other breathing-related disorders such as asthma may improve.

What you need: For this pose, you need 4 foam blocks, blankets, an area of wall space and a chair.

What you do: Support under the shoulders is very important, using either a large folded blanket or the foam blocks to avoid straining the neck. Place your blocks about 60–75cm/2–2½ feet from the wall and lie with your buttocks against the wall, your legs extending up it (Viparita Karani). Ensure that your shoulders and neck are supported by the blankets or blocks and that the back of your head is on the floor. Position the chair so that its legs are just behind your head and the seat is above you.

Walk your legs up the wall and place your hands on your lower back, as you bend your knees and move your chest towards your chin, taking the hands up your back as you do so. When the legs are vertical, lower them down on to the chair. You may find the height of the seat itself is a little low – a couple of folded

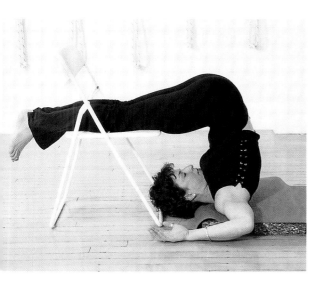

blankets will make it more comfortable and supportive for the lower back. Once you are in Halasana, the arms can be taken over the head to release the shoulders fully, and the posture can be held for 5 minutes or more. Come out of the posture slowly and carefully, and rest in a sitting-forward bend with legs crossed in front of you (Sukhasana) or extended out in front, keeping your spine upright (Paschimottanasana). Hold for 8 breaths.

How long? Hold for 20 breaths.

Top Tip: Avoid this posture during menstruation or if you have high blood pressure.

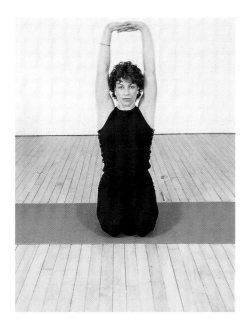

Kneeling With Shoulder Release (Urdhva Baddha Hastasana)

What it does: Relieves stiffness and discomfort in the shoulders and the neck. Helps to lengthen the spine and improve areas of tightness. Therapeutic for symptoms of osteoarthritis in the shoulders.

What you do: Sit either with legs crossed in Sukhasana, if you find this position comfortable, or alternatively sit on your heels. Ensure the spine is lifting and upright.

Bring your hands in towards your chest and interlock the fingers firmly. Extend the palms and the arms away from you. Open out into the corners of the chest to lengthen the neck and move the shoulders back and down.

Extend the arms from their position parallel to the floor up towards the ceiling, bringing the creases of the elbows towards each other and the upper arms towards the ears. Continue to maintain length between the ears and the shoulders and ensure the head remains centrally positioned over the spine with the back of the neck long. Hold for at least 6 breaths with one hand position and then repeat by placing the other index finger on top when you interlace the fingers and extend the arms away again. Rest forward with your bottom on your heels, forehead to the floor, arms alongside legs with palms to the ceiling (Balasana, or child pose).

How long? Hold for 8–10 breaths.

lifestyle workouts

We spend more and more of our day sitting down. Are you sitting with good posture? Have you ever wondered whether your sitting position could be contributing to your stiff back or sore knees or even just limited mobility? Here is a quick guide to get your body in the right position.

Are you sitting comfortably?

Symmetry

First take a look at your knee position. Ideally the angle at the hip and at the knees should not be less than 90°. To help you achieve this, make sure that you keep your knees directly over your feet, and that your feet are not tucked underneath the chair. If you have a smaller angle at your hips then you will be creating more lumbar flexion, which puts more pressure on the vertebra discs. If the angle at the hips is greater than 90°, this will put your spine into lumbar extension, causing the lumbar spine to be flatter, which is much better for posture.

Solution

To help you correct your lumbar position you can use a lumbar roll. These are excellent – simply roll up a hand towel and stuff it in an old pair of tights and then tie it round the back of your chair to keep it in the right position.

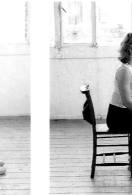

Sitting with good posture

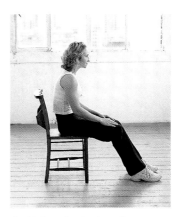

Try to avoid excessive leaning forward.

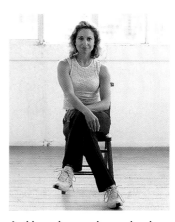

Avoid slumping backwards.

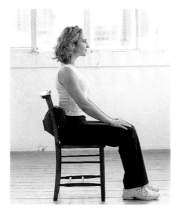

Using a lumbar roll can help to correct posture.

Alternatively you can secure your towel with two elastic bands to keep the roll tight and in place. Ensure your weight is distributed evenly on each leg. Avoid crossing your legs, as this pushes your spine into a diagonal curve.

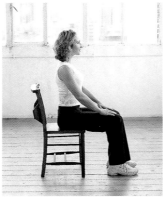

Avoid crossing your legs, or leaning on one hip.

Office Workout

If you find yourself chained to your desk for hours on end, and despair at not being able to improve your body and reduce the stresses of your day, this workout is for you. It will relieve the muscle tension often felt in the upper body and stored in the lower spine and sacrum area, and correct muscle imbalances caused by sitting for prolonged periods. It will also address the problem areas of hips and thighs. And just because you are sitting down you don't have to forego flattening those abdominals.

The Workout

Shoulder Roll x 8

Seated Spine Rotation x 4, right and left

Slumped Hamstring Stretch x 1, right and left

Chest Stretch x 1

Alternate Neck Stretch x 1

Seated Abdominal Work x 8

Seated Spine Rotation x 4, right and left

Slumped Hamstring Stretch, right and left

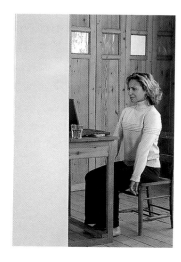
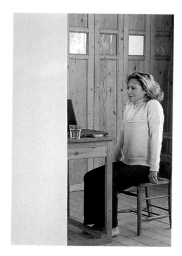
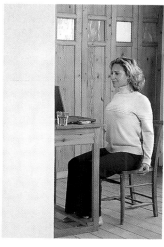
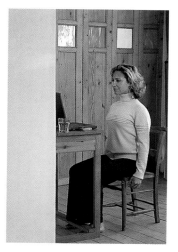

Shoulder Roll

What it does: Loosens the shoulders and relieves tension.

What you do: Draw a circle with your shoulders, lifting them towards your ears, back down your spine and then forwards. Repeat, reversing the direction of your circle.

How many? At least 8.

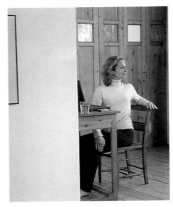
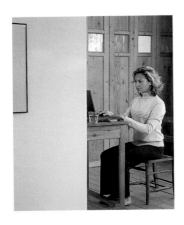

Seated Spine Rotation

What it does: Releases tension in the middle back.

What you do: Sit up tall on a chair. Your feet need to be flat on the floor and directly under your knees. Place your right hand on the outside of your left thigh and reach back with your left hand. Be tall as you turn. You can use your hands as levers to increase the stretch you feel. Only stretch to a comfortable position, holding for 10–15 seconds, and repeat on the other side.

How many? Build up to 8

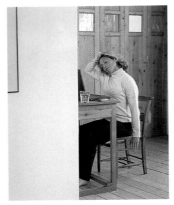
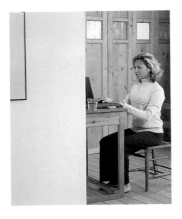

Alternate Neck Stretch

What it does: This is good for relieving muscle tension in the neck, and an excellent stress minimizer. Eastern cultures believe a great deal of our stress resides in the neck.

What you do: Sit with good posture, neck long and shoulders relaxed. Tilt your right ear towards your right shoulder. Keep the shoulders level. Place the right hand on the side of the left ear and gently press down. Extend the left hand away from your head. You should feel a stretch in the side of the neck. To increase the stretch, hold the position and direct your head to look under your armpit. Repeat on the other side.

How long? Hold for 10–30 seconds.

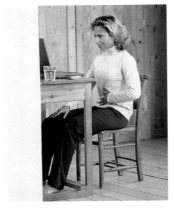
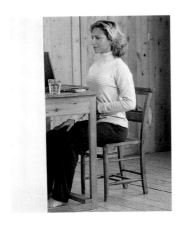

Seated Abdominal Work

What it does: Flattens, tones and supports trunk muscles.

What you do: Sit forward in your chair so your knees are over your ankles. Extend up through the spine and contract the abdominals. Draw the breast bone and the pelvic bone closer together, flexing your spine into a letter C as you contract. Hold for 30 seconds, breathe and relax.

How many? Try to do 4 every hour.

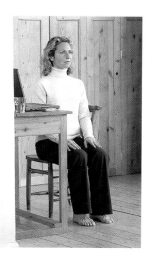 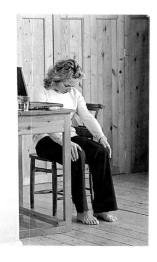 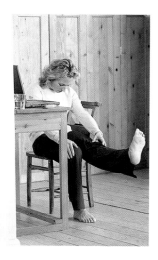

Slumped Hamstring Stretch

What it does: The hamstrings get very tight when you are sitting down, and this can pull on the lower spine and cause sciatic pain. This exercise stretches the hamstrings but also stimulates the nervous system to encourage greater relaxation in the muscle.

What you do: Sit forward in your chair, back extended. Now slump down, arching the spine and letting the shoulders hollow. Extend one leg forwards, holding the leg behind the knee. Keep slumped as you stretch the straight leg away from you. You may feel some tingling in your upper back. This is not uncommon and is caused by the stimulation of the nerve endings in your shoulders.

How long? Hold for 30 seconds.

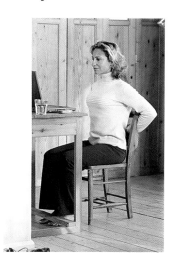

Chest Stretch

What it does: When you are reading documents or working away at a computer the shoulders tend to draw in and rise. This stretch counteracts this and helps to open up the shoulder area.

What you do: Sit slightly forward in your chair. Link your hands behind your body, drawing the shoulder blades together.

How long? Hold for 10 –30 seconds.

Wall Workout

Sometimes we can try too hard to be creative with our workouts. The Wall Workout keeps things really simple, whilst ensuring that your body is in the right position for you to to see and feel results. All you need is yourself and a flat wall. The Exercise ball can add variety but other than that you can do this workout anywhere, anytime. It will tone your thighs, hips and buttocks, strengthen your trunk muscles, flatten your abdominals, stimulate vital strength in your upper body and improve the mobility of your spine.

Body Kit
Small block
Exercise ball or basket ball/football

The Workout
Wall Roll-Down x 8
Wall Touch x 8, right and left
Inner Thigh Press x 16, right and left
Inclined Press-up x 12
Exercise Ball Roll-down x 16
Inclined Triceps Press-up x 12
Back Lift x 8
Standing Glut Ballet Lift x 16, right and left

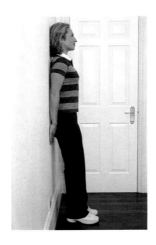
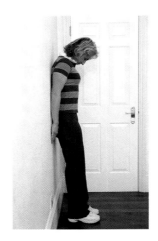
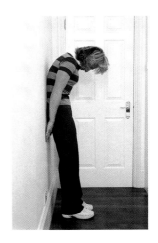
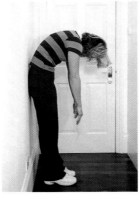
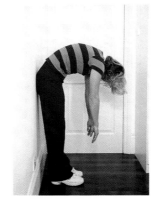

Wall Roll-down

What it does: A great way to mobilize the spine.

What you do: Stand with your back against a wall. Ensure that all of your back is in contact with the wall. You may need to be about 30cm/12in away from the wall to ensure your lumbar spine is touches it. Slowly, one vertebra at a time, peel off the wall, starting with your head, until you reach your tail bone. Use your abdominals to control your movement and to encourage your spine to flex. Then slowly unravel and peel yourself back up the wall, ensuring all parts of the spine come in contact with the wall as you uncurl. Breathe smoothly throughout.

How many? Up to 8

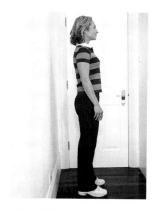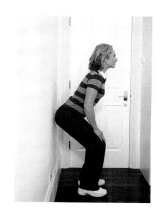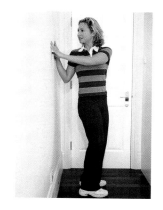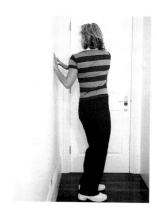

Wall Touch

What it does: Improves the mobility of the spine and tones the waist.

What you do: Stand with your back to the wall, about 30cm/12in away from it. Maintaining good posture, perform a small squat, extend up through the body and rotate your body towards the wall, aiming to touch it with your hand. Concentrate on keeping the hips facing the front. Draw in through the abdominals to help you achieve this. Face the front again, repeat the squat, extend and rotate in the other direction.

How many? 8 on each side

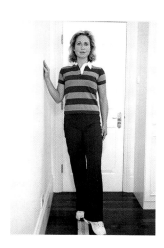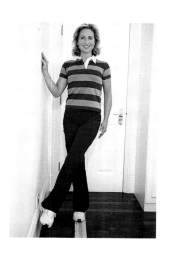

Inner Thigh Press

What it does: Tones the inner thigh.

What you do: Stand on a small block or stair sideways to the wall. Extend the outside leg forwards, rotate the leg at the hip to expose the inner thigh to the ceiling, extend the leg and then slightly soften it at the knee whilst keeping the original length of the leg – important as it helps to lengthen the leg as you work. This is your start position. Press the leg from the inner thigh across the standing leg, and focus on 'scooping' the inner thigh as you lift. This engages the inner thigh muscle more. Return to the starting position. Make sure you pull up through the body as you support yourself.

How many? 16 on each side

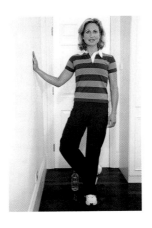
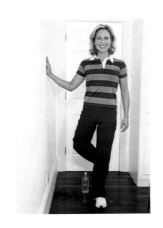

Standing Glut Ballet Lift

What it does: Lifts the gluteal muscles.

What you do: Stand sideways to the wall, about 30cm/12in away from it. Maintaining good posture, lift your right leg, opening at the hip. Your right knee should be pointing towards the wall and the foot directly behind the supporting ankle. This is your start position. Now extend the bent leg back, keeping the knee pointing towards the wall. Draw the working leg back in behind the supporting ankle as in the start position. Repeat on the other leg.

How many? 16

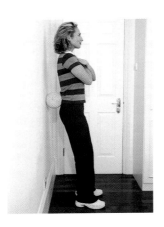
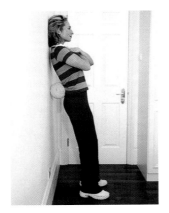

Back Lift

What it does: Strengthens the back extensor muscles.

What you do: Stand with your back to the wall and place a small ball in the lower part of your spine. Cross your arms, resting your fingertips on your shoulders, contract the abdominals and pull up through the pelvic floor muscles. Slowly lean back from the hips to touch your shoulders gently against the wall. Only go as far as you feel comfortable doing. Come back to an upright position.

How many? 8

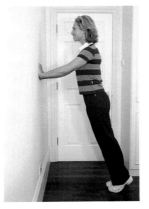
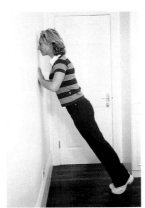

Inclined Triceps Press-up

What it does: Tightens the triceps muscle.

What you do: Place your hands on the wall a little lower than shoulder level, with the thumb and first fingers touching to form a trapezius. The elbows should be wide. Angle your body away from the wall so that your weight is on your hands. Slowly lower yourself down towards the wall as the elbows bend to the sides. Push yourself back up to a straight-arm position.

How many? 12–16

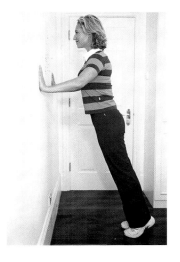
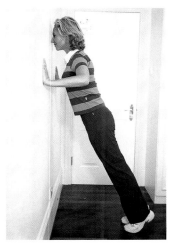

Inclined Press-up (wide arm)

What it does: Tones the chest area.

What you do: Place your hands more than shoulder-distance apart on the wall. Angle the body away from the wall and rise up on your toes. Take your weight on your hands. The further away from the wall you are, the more challenging this is. Lower the body towards the wall, keeping the abdominals tight and the hips in line.

How many? 12–16

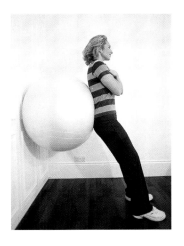
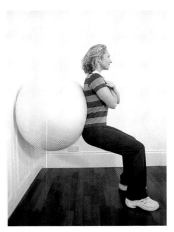

Exercise Ball Roll-down

What it does: Strengthens and tones the buttocks and thighs.

What you do: Place an exercise ball between your back and the wall. Slowly roll the ball down the wall as you squat. Keep the knees over the ankles and the abdominals contracted. Roll the ball up the wall as you come back to your starting position.

How many? 16

Car Workout

You may spend hours behind the wheel, so if you can spare a few moments when your car is parked to do this simple workout, you will help relieve tension, correct muscle imbalances and safeguard the integrity of your spine. Whether you are waiting for the children to come out of school, have a couple of minutes spare before going into a meeting or before you switch on the ignition, take the time to do this workout.

Body Kit
Ball or rolled-up newspaper

The Workout
First do the Seated Symmetry Test on page 174.

Shoulder Roll x 8 (see page 175)
Steering Wheel Shoulder Retraction x 8
Seated Spine Rotation x 4, right and left
Buttock Clench x 12
Knee Pull x 8, right and left
Inner Thigh Squeeze x 12
Steering Wheel Shoulder retraction x 8
Hip Hitch, x 8 right and left

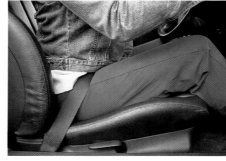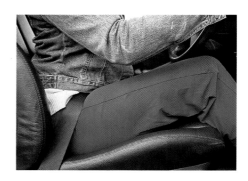

Hip Hitch

What it does: Strengthens the oblique abdominals and helps to stabilize the pelvis.

What you do: Sit with good posture. Extend up through the spine. Focus on lifting one hip up towards the ribs. Hold for 10 seconds and release. Repeat on the other side.

How many? 8 on each side

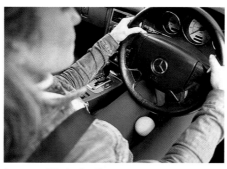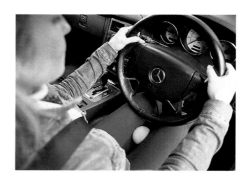

Inner Thigh Squeeze

What it does: Encourages correct positioning of the knees and reduces the risk of knee pain.

What you do: Sit with good posture. Place a ball or rolled-up newspaper between your knees and squeeze it to engage the inner thighs. Hold for 10 seconds.

How many? 12–16

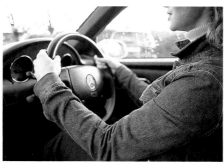
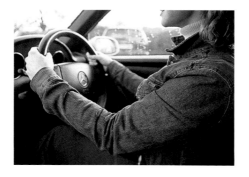

Steering Wheel Shoulder Retraction

What it does: Relieves tension in the shoulders.

What you do: Place your hands lightly on the steering wheel and pull back through the shoulders as if squeezing a lemon between your shoulder blades. Hold for 10 seconds.

How many? 8–12

Knee Pull

What it does: Encourages mobility around the sciatic hip joints.

What you do: This is only a small movement. Pull one knee towards your chest, tucking the chin into your chest. Keep the abdominals contracted as you lift the knee.

How many? 8 on each side

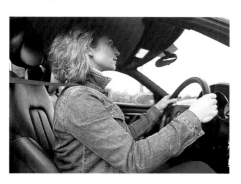
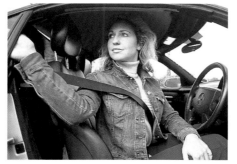

Seated Spine Rotation

What it does: Releases tension in the middle back.

What you do: Sit up tall. Your feet need to be flat on the floor and directly below your knees. Place your left hand on the outside of your right thigh and reach back with your right hand. Be tall as you turn. You can use your hands as levers to increase the stretch you feel. Stretch only to a comfortable position, holding for 10–15 seconds, and repeat on the other side.

How many? 4 on each side

Buttock Clench

What it does: Helps release tension on the sciatic nerve.

What you do: Draw the buttock cheeks together. Hold for 10 seconds and release.

How many? 12

Workout in a Suitcase

If you live your life out of a suitcase, this portable workout is for you.

Body Kit

Resistance band

Mat

Chair

The Workout

Frontal Arm Raise x 12

Outer Thigh Press x 12, right and left

Abdominal Curl with Resistance Band x 16

Side Lateral Raise x 8, right and left

Buttock Raise x 20, right and left

Shoulder Fall x 5 (hold 10 seconds each rep)

Inner Thigh Lift x 16, right and left

Chest Press x 12

Shoulder Opening x 12

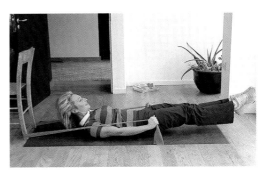

Abdominal Curl With Resistance Band

What it does: Flattens abdominal muscles.

What you do: Wrap a resistance band around bed or chair legs. Lie on your back and hold on to the resistance band ends. Curl up, leading from the breastbone, extending the legs out straight and drawing the arms in to the sides of the body. Lower slowly down. Keep your hands by your sides as you lift.

How many? 16

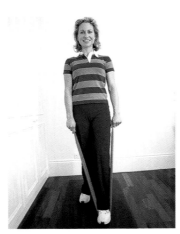

Side Lateral Raise

What it does: Tones and shapes deltoid shoulder muscle.

What you do: Maintaining good posture, stand with feet about 30cm/12in apart. Stand on the middle of the resistance band with your front foot. Hold the resistance band at both ends and adjust its length so the working arm can feel some tension on the band. Raise your arm out to the side, keeping the palm down to the floor. Check that your wrist stays in a neutral position and the body remains tall and in good alignment. Repeat with the other arm.

How many? 8–16 on each side

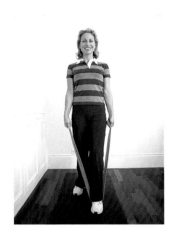
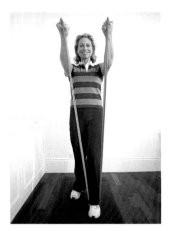

Frontal Arm Raise

What it does: Shapes the front of the shoulder and tones the long head of the biceps.

What you do: Stand with good posture, your feet 30cm/12in apart. Place your front foot on the resistance band. Hold an end of the resistance band in each hand, palms in front of the thighs, away from the body. Check that you have some tension in the band before you lift. Keeping the back straight and the abdominals contracted, lift the arms to eye level. Keep a slight bend at the elbow. Slowly lower down.

How many? 12

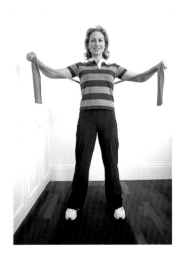
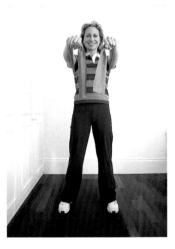

Chest Press

What it does: Helps to tone the muscles of the upper chest.

What you do: Stand with good posture. Place the resistance band around the upper back and under the armpits. Hold the ends of the band, adjusting its length by wrapping it around your hands to maintain tension. Keeping the elbows slightly bent, draw the arms in to the centre of the body, leading with the hands. Imagine you are putting your arms round a barrel as you do this, and then return to the starting position. If you look in the mirror as you do this exercise, you should see the chest being lifted as your elbows squeeze together. The movement should be slow and controlled.

How many? 12–16

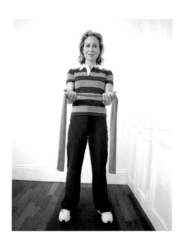

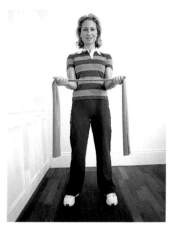

Shoulder Opening

What it does: Tones the muscles of the upper back. Make a special effort to do this exercise if you are round-shouldered or spend a lot of time working on the computer keyboard.

What you do: Stand with good posture. Hold the resistance band in front of you. Keep your elbows tucked in to your sides, forearms at 90°, hands shoulder-distance apart. Keeping your elbows close to your sides, pull the band away from the mid-line of the body. Try to create as large a distance as possible between your hands. Return to the starting position with control.

How many? 12

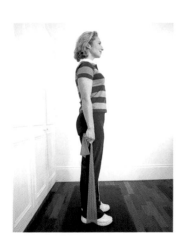

Shoulder Fall

What it does: Excellent for improving posture and stopping your shoulders creeping up around your ears!

What you do: Stand with both feet on the middle of the resistance band, and hold an end in each hand. Position your feet wide enough apart so when you stand up there is some tension in your band. With this exercise (unlike the others) try to minimize the tension in the band by letting it ease your shoulders away from your ears.

How many? 8

Top Tip: As you get more proficient with this exercise, practice your Kegal exercises (see page 147) at the same time.

Inner Thigh Lift

What it does: Helps streamline the inner thigh.

What you do: Tie the resistance band around your ankles, so that it forms a loop about 30cm/12in in length. Lie on your side. Bring your top leg in front of you on to the floor. The other leg should be stretched out along the floor. The loop of the resistance

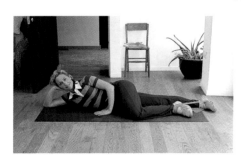

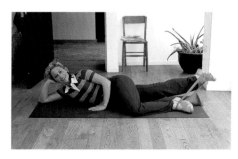

band should be resting across the top of your laces (top leg) and under the sole of your foot (bottom leg). You may need to adjust the loop size. Keeping the top leg firmly on the floor, lift and lower the bottom leg. Focus on lifting from the inner thigh. Make sure you keep the foot and the knee of this leg facing forwards. The resistance band needs to be kept taut throughout.

How many? 16–20

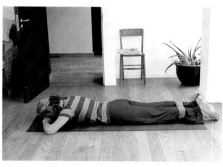 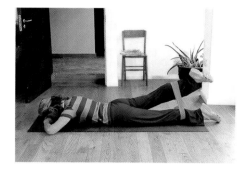

Buttock Raise

What it does: This exercise will really lift your buttock cheeks.

What you do: Keep the resistance band tied around the ankles (as in the Inner Thigh Lift exercise). Lie face down, with your forehead resting on your hands. Raise one leg, keeping your hips on the floor, and lengthen the leg as you lift from the buttocks. Slowly lower the leg back down to the floor. Repeat with the other leg. Build up to 20 reps.

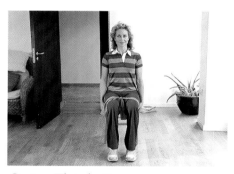 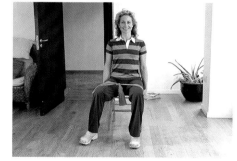

Outer Thigh Press

What it does: Tones and streamlines the outer thighs.

What you do: Sit on a chair, maintaining good posture. Tie a resistance band around your thighs. Ensure there is tension in the band before you start. Slowly take one thigh out to the side, then return it to the centre position. Keep your back straight throughout the whole exercise. Repeat with the other thigh.

How many? 12–20 on each side

Aeroplane Workout

I have sequenced this workout using a concept called peripheral heat action (PHA). This technique helps to stimulate blood circulation by encouraging the blood to move from the upper to the lower body in succession. This is particularly helpful when exercising in a restricted space.

The workout

Shoulder Roll x 8

Upper Back Stretch x 1

Seated spine Rotation x 1, right and left

Toe Crunches Forward x 4

Toe crunches Backward x 4

Overhead Press x 4

Single Knee Pull x 8, left and right

Toe Crunch Forward x 4

Toe Crunch Backward x 4

Overhead Press x 4

Single Knee Pull x 8, left and right

Upper Back Stretch x 1

Seated Spine Rotation x 1, right and left

Shoulder Roll x 8

Top tip

Aim to take some gentle walking exercise for 20 minutes before and after the flight.

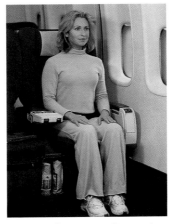
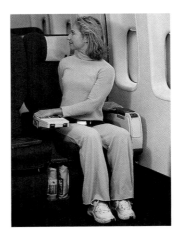

Seated Spine Rotation

What it does: Stretches the shoulders, chest and upper back. Rotating the body will increase the mobility of the spine.

What you do: Sit forward in your seat, with your knees directly over your ankles, back straight, abdominals contracted and spine extended. Place your left hand across and in front of your body, holding on to the right arm rest. Place the right arm behind you, reaching towards the left arm rest. If you can, hold on to both arm rests. Feel a stretch across the upper chest and shoulders as you extend tall. Change sides. To develop this stretch, rotate your body to the right when the left hand is front of the body and rotate the body to the left when the right hand is in front. Hold for 10–30 seconds each side.

How many? 8 on both sides

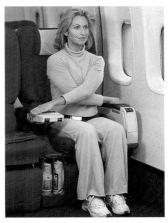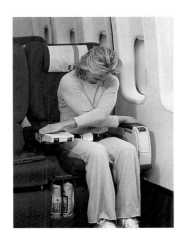

Upper Back Stretch

What it does: Stretches the trapezius and rhomboids (the stress-holding muscles between the shoulder blades). Great for tension sufferers!

What you do: Cross both arms in front of your body and hold on to the arm rests with a firm grip. Pull inwards with both hands, and at the same time extend through the spine. Lowering the chin to the chest will increase the stretch felt across the upper back.

How long? Hold for 10–30 seconds.

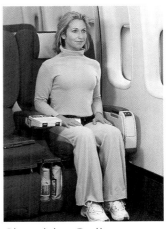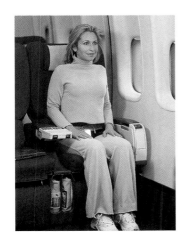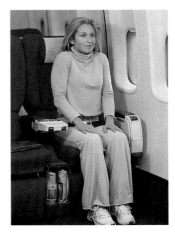

Shoulder Roll

What it does: Loosens the houlders and relieves tension.

What you do: Draw a circle with your shoulders, lifting them towards your ears, back down your spine and then forwards. Reverse.

How many? 8 in either direction

Overhead Press

What it does: Increases mobility and stimulates blood circulation towards upper body. With weights (hand weights or filled water bottles), this exercise can help to strengthen the upper arms.

What you do: Start with your hands on your thighs. Lift your hands up to your shoulders and then press your hands directly over the head. Lower the hands back down to the thighs.

How much? 12

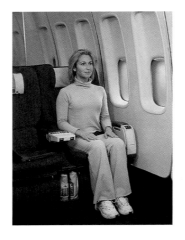 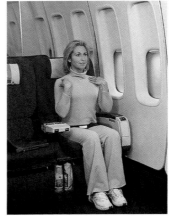 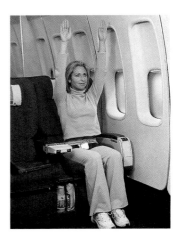

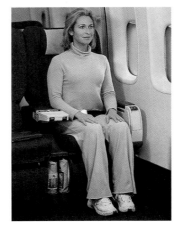 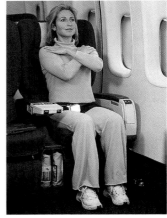

Back Extension

What it does: Strengthens the back extensor muscles.

What you do: Sit forward in your seat, keep your knees directly over your ankles and your back straight. Cross your arms over your chest with your fingertips resting on your shoulders. Pulling in your abdominals, lean back so your shoulders touch the seat. Come back to an upright position.

How many? 8–12

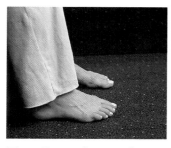 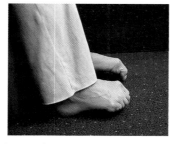 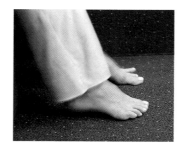

Toe Crunches – forwards and backwards

What it does: Encourages blood circulation in the feet and legs. Strengthens the arch of the foot, which can become weak and put pressure on the knees.

What you do: With your shoes off, sit with good posture, your feet tucked under your knees. Curl your toes up towards your heels, as if trying to pick something up with them. Relax the toes. Repeat, but this time keep the toes drawn in as you reach back with the heels to stretch out the feet.

How many? 10 in both directions

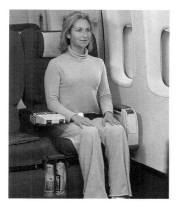 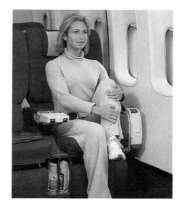 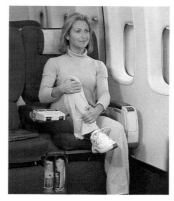

Single Knee Pulls

What it does: Encourages blood circulation to the legs.

What you do: Slowly lift one leg in to your chest. Hold the leg gently at the knee and across the shin. Beware of pulling the knee in too tightly if you have knee problems. Lower down and repeat on the other side.

How many? 8–12 on each leg

Hotel Workout

Travelling need not throw your regular exercise routine into turmoil. This workout has been designed for a small space.

Body Kit

Pillow

Resistance band.

The Workout

Seated Sun Salutation x 4

Seated Spine Rotation x 4, right and left

Wall Bridges x 8

Abdominal Pillow Roll x8, right and left

Bed Toe-touch x 8

Prone Pillow Leg Lift x 8

Resistance Band Lateral Raise x 12

Triceps Dip x 12

Abdominal Curl with Resistance Band x 12 (see page 184)

Seated Sun Salutation x 4

Optional Extras

Complement cardio goals with:

Walking. Don't forget to pack your pedometer – walking is a great way to build in some cardiovascular benefits when away from home.

The mobility workout (see page 99) to help relieve stiffness.

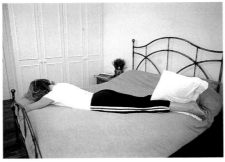

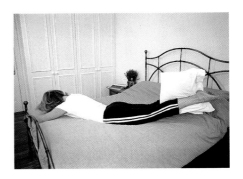

Prone Pillow Leg Lift

What it does: Tightens the buttocks and lower back extensor muscles.

What you do: Lie face down, on the bed or floor. Place a pillow between your feet. Engage your abdominals to support the spine. Slowly lengthen the legs and squeeze the pillow as you lift them off the floor. Slowly lower back down.

How many? 8–12

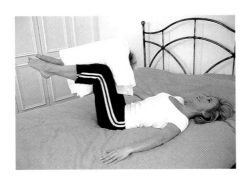

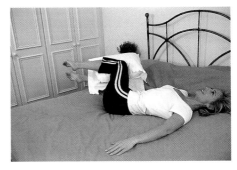

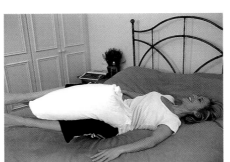

Abdominal Pillow Roll

What it does: Develops trunk stability of the abdominals and tones the waist muscles.

What you do: Lie on the bed or floor, knees bent and feet down flat. Place a pillow or cushion between your knees, then lower them to one side. As you draw the knees back to a central position, concentrate on contracting the abdominals down to the floor, thereby stimulating the oblique abdominal girdle to contract and tighten the waist. Repeat on other side.

How many? 8–12 each side

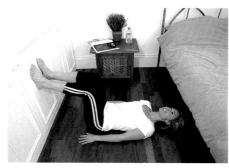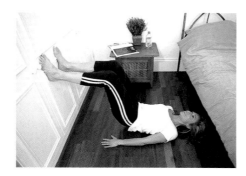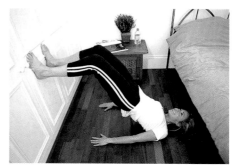

Wall Bridge

What it does: Mobilizes the spine, tightens the buttocks and improves trunk stability.

What you do: Lie on your back on the floor with your knees bent at 90° and feet on the wall. Contracting the abdominals, tilt the pelvis as you peel off the floor, raising your body on to your shoulders. Keep the hips level and abdominals contracted to support the spine. Roll down the spine to the floor position.

How many? 8

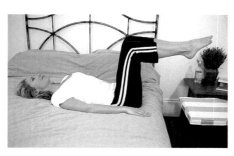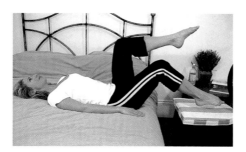

Bed Toe-touch

What it does: Targets the lower abdominals.

What you do: Place a chair about 30cm/12in away from the bed. Lie on the bed, on your back, with your bottom towards the edge. Pre-contract your abdominals. Slowly lower one leg down to the chair, then draw it slowly back again. Repeat on the other side. This is a challenging exercise. The further the chair is from the bed, the more challenging the exercise is for the abdominals. If you are new to the exercise, just lower your toes down to the bed and progress to the chair.

How many? 8–12 on each leg

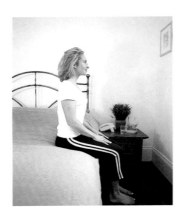
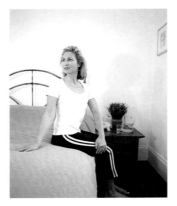

Seated Spine Rotation

What it does: Mobilizes the spine – great to do first thing in the morning when getting out of bed.

What you do: Sit on the side of your bed with your back straight and knees over your ankles. Keep the hips and knees facing forwards, and place your left hand on the outside of your right thigh. Place your right hand behind your back with the palm on the bed. Rotate your back to the right, so that you aim to look behind you. Make sure you pull up tall, for this will protect your spine as you rotate.

How many? 4–6

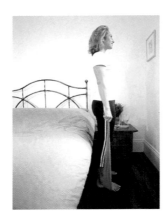
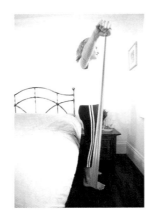

Resistance Band Lateral Raise

What it does: Tones the deltoid muscle of the shoulders.

What you do: Stand on a resistance band. Hold the resistance band in each hand. Maintaining good posture, lift the resistance band to the side, level with the shoulders. Keep the palms facing down to the floor as you lift. Once the band is level with the shoulders, rotate the hands so the palms face up, then rotate the palms down and slowly lower back down to the floor.

How many? 12

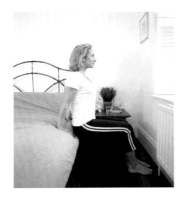
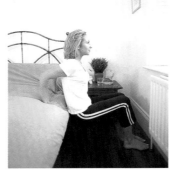

Triceps Dip

What it does: Tightens the back of the arm.

What you do: Sit on side of your bed or the bath, hands hip-distance apart and fingertips facing your toes. Lift your body weight off the bed or bath and lower yourself to the floor, bending at the elbow. Make sure the elbows stay pointing towards the back wall. Extend the arm straight, keeping your back close to the edge. The further the feet are away from the bed or bath, the harder this exercise is.

How many? 12–16

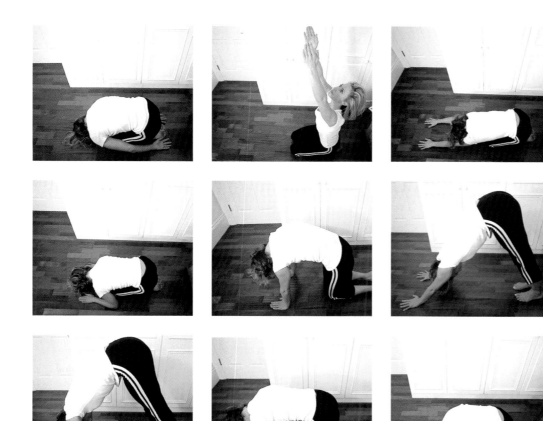

Seated Sun Salutation

What it does: Aids relaxation, lengthens the spine and hamstrings.

What you do: Kneel on the floor or bed, arms by your sides, resting your chest on your knees. Sweep your fingers along the floor as you extend your arms up towards the ceiling. Next, reach forward with your arms and extend through your fingers, so that you feel the stretch through the whole arm as you reach out with your hands. Draw your hands back by your shoulders and push up into a box position, wrists under shoulders, hips over knees. Spread your fingers and tuck your toes underneath you. Take the weight on your hands and push your hips high feeling a stretch along the spine and chest area as you press your heels to the floor. Take 4 deep breaths in this position. Lift up on to your toes taking your weight on to the upper body as you lower your knees to the floor. Come back into the box position and finish in the start pose. Repeat 4 times.

Playtime Workout

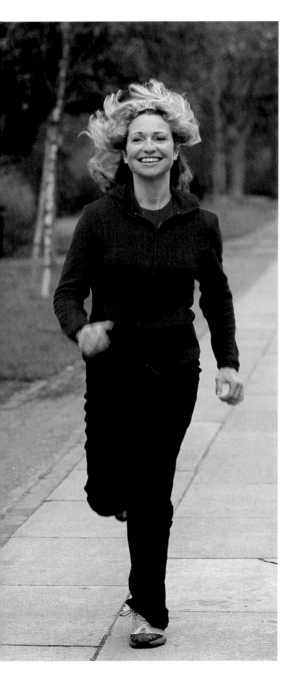

It may be grey and cold outside, but that's no reason to neglect your fitness. Turn the cold weather into your friend. The chilly weather can boost your metabolic rate by up to 40%, as the body has to work to maintain its internal temperature. And if it's snowing, even better – half an hour of brisk snow-walking burns 366 calories – 3 times more than you'd burn on bare ground. So what are you waiting for? Get outside, enjoy being active – whatever the weather, have a laugh and burn those calories!

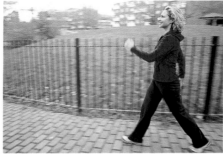

Start with a warm-up

Walk at a brisk pace until you feel your muscles start to loosen. You will need to go a little further in cold weather (5–10 minutes).

The Workout

Begin the workout with a 5–10-minute bout of cardio. Here are some options:

- Sprint to the top of a hill
- Run a slalom course through trees or signposts
- Power-jump over a mound of leaves or low bench
- Kick a football across a park
- Run a relay between park benches

Next, mix in one of the following 5 drills (each takes 2–4 minutes). After each drill, immediately do another round of cardio. Complete the cardio-drill cycle at least 3 times in each workout for the best results.

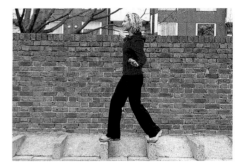

Walk The Plank

What it does: Challenges balance and the deep core stability muscles.

What you do: Simply find a sturdy fence, curb or wide beam, and hop on it! Take each step slowly and with control, stabilize yourself by keeping your abdominals tight. Hold the abdominal contraction as you walk. Don't worry if your balance is not too good to start – it will improve with practice.

Tree Presses

What it does: Tones the ectoral muscles of the chest.

What you do: Find yourself a sturdy fence, tree or post and do some slow press-ups against it.

Repeat 10–20 times.

Firm Your Backside

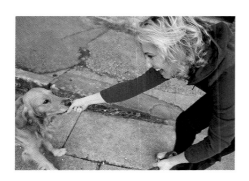

What it does: Firms all muscles of the hips and thighs.

What you do: Be creative with your walking! Try a series of walking lunges or a slow-motion uphill power-walk. The incline will increase your calorie burn.

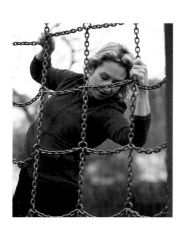

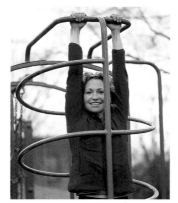

Build Back Strength

What it does: Strengthens the back, shoulder and arm muscles.

What you do: Reach for a low branch and use your arms and back muscles to pull yourself up. If this is too tough, jump into the pull-up position and slowly lower yourself to the ground. Controlling the ease-down is the key element in improving your strength. Do as many as you can.

Involve The Kids

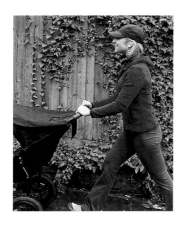

What it does: Strengthens your back muscles while achieving a cardio benefit.

What you do: Don't let the children stop you getting fit – involve them. Load them on their pushchair or tricycles, or scooters and get moving. If you are using a sledge, keep your arms straight as you pull it behind you – and for extra resistance, head for a gentle uphill slope. Or simply pull your sledge or baby buggy towards you with a rowing motion (great for your back). Remember to pull safely, you need to use your upper back muscles and contract your abdominals to protect your back.

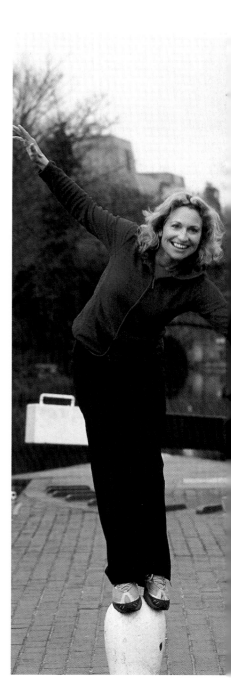

Don't Panic! Plan

The Plan

Do 2 sets of 20 repetitions for each exercise. Do the programme 3 times a week, resting a day between workouts. You have two options: you can follow the home plan or do it in the gym – wherever you feel most comfortable. Everybody can do the same number of sets and repetitions, but adjust the weight according to your fitness level – however do remember to reach your point of near fatigue for each exercise.

Warm-up

Warm up for 5–10 minutes with light cardiovascular work, either on cardiovascular equipment in your gym or with a brisk walk or jog outside. Make sure you move your arms to get a full-body warm-up.

Cool-down

Cool down with 5 minutes of light aerobic work, followed by stretches for all your major muscle groups (see page 129). Remember to hold each stretch for 20–30 seconds without bouncing.

Optional Extras

For a flat tummy, don't forget your abs! Aim to do 3 sets of the Abdominal Best Body Bits (see page 77) 3 times a week. These can either be done at the same time as your Build a Beach Body Workout or on your rest days.

If you need to shed some excess winter body fat, supplement the programme with your daily pedometer walking targets (see page 44) and a minimum of 30 minutes' structured cardio exercise 3 times a week.

Build a Beach Body in 4 Weeks Flat!

If you have taken it a little too easy in spring and the summer holiday is fast approaching, this workout is for you. There is still time to get your body into shape and feel confident in your swimsuit. So, what are you waiting for? Be Active!

These exercises have been designed to work a combination of muscles simultaneously – the end result? Better results in less time! I have used equipment in a gym, but each exercise has a home option so you don't need to miss out!

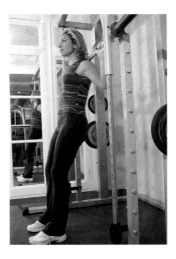 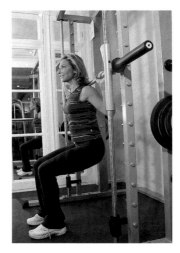

GYM: Squat

What it does: Works the gluteals, hamstrings and quads. This exercise targets the buttocks and tops of the thighs.

What you do: Adjust the Smith Machine so that the bar is at shoulder height. Release the locks and hold the bar with your hands slightly wider than your shoulders, so the bar rests across the shoulders and upper back. Place your feet about hip-distance apart, slightly forward of the bar; keep the abdominals contracted and chest lifted. Your legs should be straight but not locked at the knee. Keep your weight in the heels of your feet. Using your legs, push up to the starting position.

Weight range: No added weight.

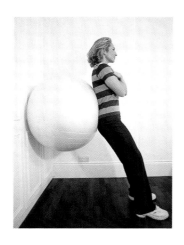
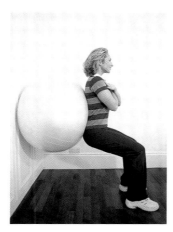

HOME: Exercise Ball Squat

What you do: Place an exercise ball in the lower part of your spine, supporting it between your back and the wall. Angle your legs away from the ball so your feet are a little distance away and the knee angle at 90° or a little more. Keep the weight in your heels. Slowly lower your body down the wall, bending at the knees so the thighs are parallel to the floor. Slowly push yourself back up to a straight position.

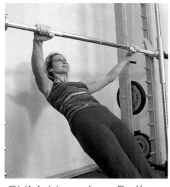
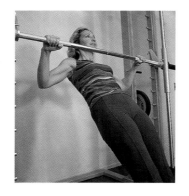
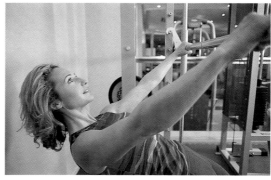

GYM: Hanging Pull-up

What it does: Strengthens the upper and middle back, shoulders and biceps.

What you do: Adjust and lock the bar on the Smith Machine to chest height. Hold the bar with your palms facing up, arms straight and hands slightly wider than shoulders. Walk forward until the legs are in a straight line and the body at an angle, in one straight line from head to toe. Use the abdominals and squeeze your shoulder blades together to maintain the position; do not let the hips drop. Bend the elbows, pulling the chest up towards the bar. Slowly straighten the arms and repeat.

Weight Range: No added weight.

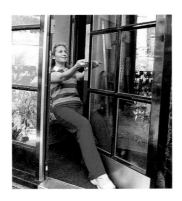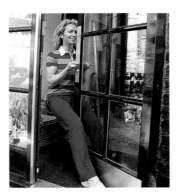

HOME: Door Pull-in

What you do: Open a door and stand with a leg on either side of the frame. Hold on to the door handles with palms up, arms extended. Keep the abdominals contracted as you pull your upper body up towards your hands. Slowly lower down.

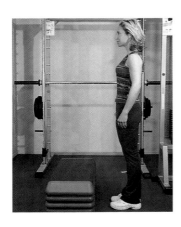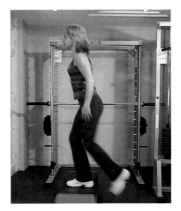

GYM: Same Leg Step Up

What it does: Tones the quadriceps, buttocks and calves, and boosts the calorie-burning effect of the workout.

What you do: Stand in front of a low flat bench, maintaining good posture. Tightening your buttocks, step up on the bench so your right leg is straight and the left foot joins the leg on the bench. Lower the left leg down to the floor and repeat. Hold dumbbells to progress in this exercise. Repeat with the other leg.

Weight Range: No weight, or up to 2.25–3.6kg/5–8lb dumbbells in each hand if advanced.

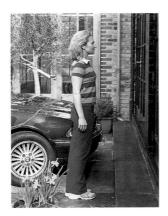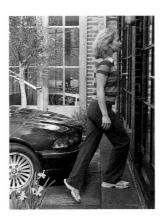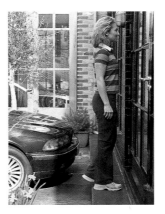

HOME: Same Leg Step-ups

What you do: Find yourself a stair, bench or step, and perform the same exercise as in the gym option.

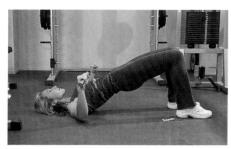 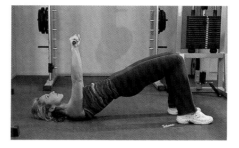

GYM: Bridge Chest Press

What it does: Shapes the shoulders, biceps and chest, and strengthens the abdominals.

What you do: Lie on your back with your knees bent and feet flat on the floor, holding dumbbells with the elbows bent at shoulder level. Tighten your buttocks and abdominals as you lift your buttocks off the floor into a bridge position. With the hips raised, press the dumbbells up over the chest, then lower weights to start. Maintain the bridge and repeat.

Weight Range: Select a weight that will ensure your chest muscles have reached near fatigue by the end of your reps.

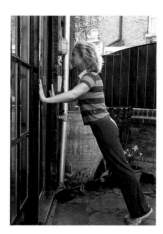 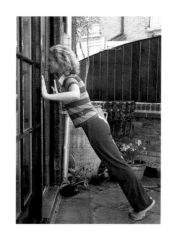

HOME: Open Door Press-up

What you do: Place your hands a little below shoulder-height on either side of an open door frame. Angle the body away from the door so you are in a straight line from the head through to the toes. Slowly lower your upper body in a straight line down towards the frame. Keep the abdominals contracted as you lower. Slowly push yourself back to a straight line. Check that your bottom stays in line with your spine.

Sore knees, aching back and painful shins may be familiar each time you exercise, but they are not inevitable. Tiresome problems such as these can be symptoms of weakness and imbalance in the key muscles that support the activities you do. The following simple moves will help to protect you from injury.

The Workout

Work up to 2 sets of 8–12 repetitions, 2–3 days a week.

Top Tips

Injuries are not an inevitable part of exercising. To prevent any possible problems, always remember to:

1. Prep-up

Do a warm-up, cool-down and stretch with each workout.

2. Get your technique right

Poor technique in repetitive sports such as tennis can cause injury quickly, so if you are having pains, do seek professional lessons as this can help you re-educate your movement patterns and decrease your risk of injury.

3. Get specific

Target the muscles you use for your sport. If you play golf, include all the muscles you use to hit a ball in your strength-training routine. But remember to train all of the major groups to achieve a balanced programme, which will reduce your risk of injury.

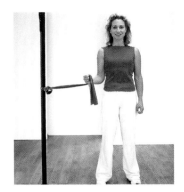
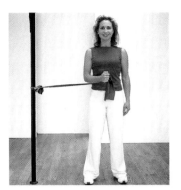
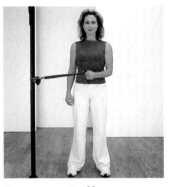
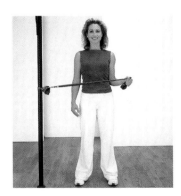

Rotator Cuff

Who should do it: Any racket sports player. Playing sports and working out can put your shoulders at risk. Strengthening the rotator cuff muscles that stabilize the joints will protect your shoulders.

What you do: Tie one end of a resistance band to a door knob. Hold the other end in your right hand. Bend your right arm so your elbow is against your side and your forearm lies across your abdomen. Remember to keep the band taut. Keeping your elbow stable, draw your hand away from your abdomen while pulling the band across the front of your body. Hold for 3 seconds, then return to the starting position. Complete a set on both sides. Then turn around, this time starting with your forearm away from your body, and with the band taut, pull it in towards your abdomen. Once you have worked the muscle in both directions, switch arms.

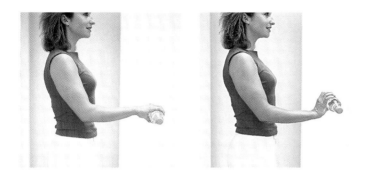

Wrist Extension

Who should do it: People who are prone to golfer's elbow and tennis elbow. Elbow pain usually comes from movements at the wrist, so strengthening the forearm muscles can prevent wrist injuries.

What you do: With your right elbow bent at your side, palm down, hold a light weight of 900g–1.35kg/2–3lb. Tilt your knuckles up towards the ceiling, hold and release. Similarly, rotate your wrist to the right and left to strengthen it in all directions. Complete a set, then switch hands.

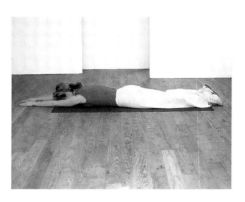
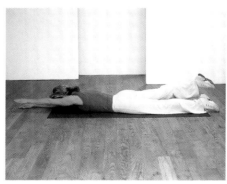

Superman

Why you should do it: Even active people can neglect lower back pain. This exercise can help strengthen the lower back and prevent injury.

What you do: Lie face-down on a mat, arms straight ahead, palms down. Raise your right arm and left leg 5cm/2in off the floor. Hold, lower, then switch sides. When that gets too easy, try lifting both legs and arms simultaneously.

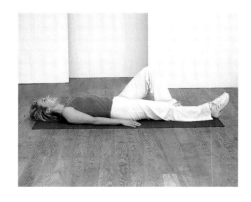
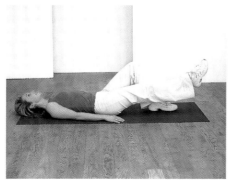

Straight Leg Lock and Lift

Why you should do it: Knee pain is extremely common. Strengthening the muscles that support the kneecap can help you avoid knee discomfort and inflammation.

What you do: Lie on your back, left leg bent, right leg straight, arms at your sides. Contract your right quadriceps gently, lock your knee, and raise your foot 15–20cm/6–8in. Hold for 5–7 seconds, then lower. Breathe comfortably throughout. Complete a set, then switch legs. When the exercise becomes too easy, add ankle weights (starting at 900g/2lb).

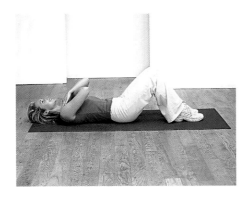 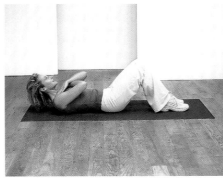

Abdominal Curl

Why you should do it: The good old abdominal curl will strengthen the abdominal wall and prevent a lot of lower back pain.

What you do: Lie flat on your back, knees bent, hands clasped behind your head or across your chest. Keeping your stomach muscles tucked in, slowly raise your shoulders off the floor about 30°. Hold and then lower.

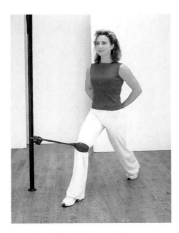 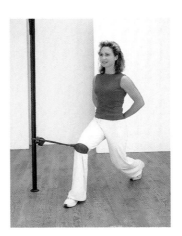

Wobbly Knee Beater

Why you should do it: Weak knees and pain around or underneath the kneecap can often be caused by an imbalance between the muscles on the inside and outside of the joint. This exercise targets the weaker medialis muscles of the quadriceps, which are attached around the inside of the knee. Strengthening these important postural muscles will benefit anyone with weak knees who is embarking on a walking or running programme.

What you do: Tie a resistance band securely around your right knee and attach it to something stable, such as table leg. Stand with your left foot behind you, your heel slightly raised. Next slowly bend your right knee, making sure it is correctly aligned over your foot. Then straighten your leg, and repeat.

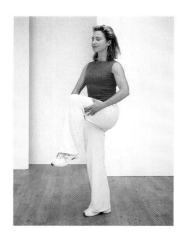

Achilles Ankle Strengthener

Why you should do it: When you are running or walking, the foot naturally tends to roll in, or pronate, with each footstrike. This may cause over-pronation and consequent pain in the Achilles tendon. This exercise will help to strengthen the Achilles tendon and encourage blood circulation to that part of the body. If you have experienced Achilles problems before, you should do this exercise as part of your warm-up.

What you do: Stand with good posture, weight even on both feet. Slowly draw your weight on to the right leg, lifting your lef leg off the floor. Close your eyes and balance for 30 seconds. Repeat on the other side. The higher you lift the supporting leg, the more challenging it is for your Achilles tendon.

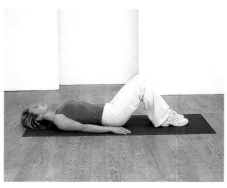
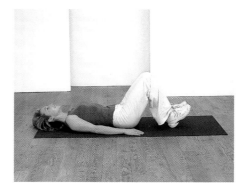

Shin Strengthener

Why you should do it: Anyone who has been power-walking on roads and hard surfaces will be familiar with the tender pain associated with shin splints – the inflammation of the anterior tibialis muscles which lie along the front of the shin. These muscles are often weak and are prone to inflammation when we increase our walking, particularly on hard surfaces where the impact forces are greater.

What you do: Lie on your back, knees bent, feet flat on the floor. Lift your toes off the floor, drawing them into your shins. The heels stay on the floor. Hold for 10 seconds and release. To make this harder you can attach a resistance band over the top of the foot and secure it against a post. As you lift your foot you will have the extra resistance of the band to work against.

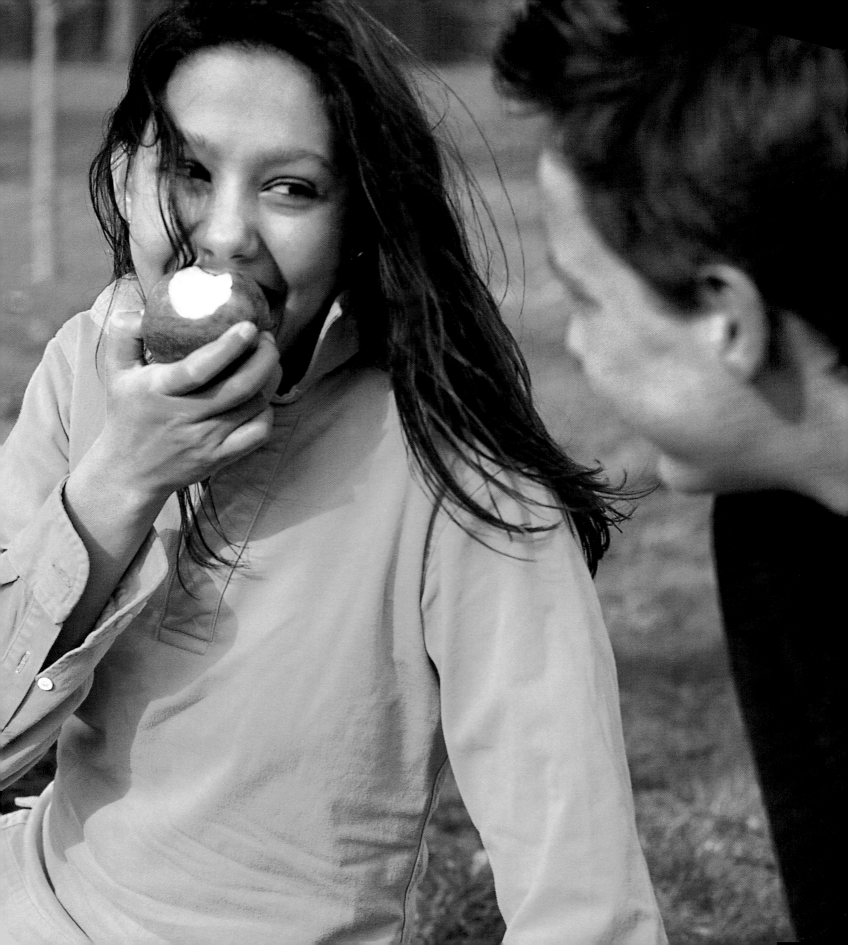

foods and fluids

Our eating habits play a fundamental part in the quality of our life and can provides us with a lot of pleasure as well as vital nutrients for good health. While training improves fitness, the results you achieve will be dependent partly on the type of foods and fluids you supply to your body. Quite simply, the condition of your body and the effectiveness of your training is directly related to the quality and quantity of the foods you consume and how well hydrated you are.

Dietary advice has become a minefield – food scares, clever marketing campaigns and complicated food labels often create confusion rather than clarity. It makes sense to eat a balanced diet, but what exactly is that? A balanced diet for someone trying to lose weight will be different from that of a serious marathon runner. No single food delivers all the nutrients the body requires to stay healthy, and a good diet should include a variety of foods from all the major food groups.

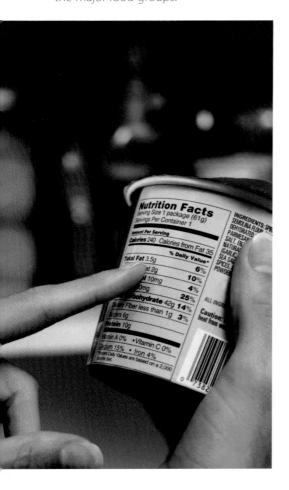

Your nutrition IQ

So just how good is your food IQ? You think you know you're eating healthily – you're counting calories and stocking up on fruit and vegetables – but are you? Do the food IQ to see if the food and drink decisions you make as you navigate your day are the best ones to boost your health and energy.

1) **Immediately you wake up, you need a quick drink to bring you round. There isn't time for breakfast, so what do you choose?**

   ☐ **a) Water**

   ☐ **b) Lashings of hot tea**

   ☐ **c) A glass of diluted orange juice**

   ⓘ Water is nutritionally 'empty', and although it's good for hydrating the body, it won't add any vitamins or minerals to your diet. One cup of tea can be good for a quick pick-me-up, but it acts as a diuretic and will make you urinate more frequently. This can lead to dehydration, especially if you don't tend to drink enough fluids anyway. More than one cup, and any benefits are soon outweighed by the disadvantages of excess caffeine. So the best choice would be diluted fruit juice. Concentrated orange juice can be so concentrated that it actually draws water from the body to help transport it across your stomach, so that not only is it being less easily absorbed, but it also potentially has fewer hydrating properties than other drinks. By diluting the juice a little you are helping to hydrate the body – essential after a night's sleep when your body naturally loses water through perspiration – and to speed up the passage of nutrients crossing the stomach lining into the body.

2) **Your weekday breakfast usually consists of:**

   ☐ **a) Toast with butter and marmalade**

   ☐ **b) A snatched Mars bar from a vending kiosk at the railway station**

   ☐ **c) Muesli with yoghurt and some fresh fruit**

   ⓘ Muesli made with oats and dried fruits contains low to moderate glycaemic index carbohydrates (see page 216), which release energy slowly right through the morning to fuel your body and your brain. Not only does the body get a better balance of nutrients to start the day, but it will also be less troubled by hunger pangs later in the morning.

   Toast, while a good source of carbohydrate (especially brown or wholemeal), does not give you as balanced a breakfast. Bread products tend to have a higher glycaemic index, which means they can initially fill us up and then leave us feeling hungry and dissatisfied as our blood sugar levels fall. Having some protein such as a poached egg with your toast will give you a better balance and help to stabilize your blood sugar level, which directly affects your energy. Complement it with a small glass of diluted OJ and you've got a more nutritionally balanced start to your day. Missing breakfast, or substituting proper food with a hastily scoffed dose of highly refined sugar is an unhealthy choice which will pick you up temporarily, but which will later leave you with a sugar 'slump' and may lead to even more unhealthy snacking. You'll find more information on top energy foods to start your day on page 224.

3) Mid-morning, you usually grab a drink of:

☐ **a) Coffee or tea, followed by water**

☐ **b) Fresh juice, and plenty of it, diluted if necessary**

☐ **c) Water**

There's nothing wrong with a cup of coffee or tea, provided you compensate for the dehydrating effects of caffeine-containing drinks by drinking plenty of water. This will also prevent too much strain being placed on the kidneys. Fresh juices are always the better option, but because they can be high in natural sugars, are best diluted. If you are watching your weight, be wary and look out for all the hidden calories these can contain. If you are getting your 8 glasses of fluid from orange juice, you could be consuming an extra 1,000 calories a day without even eating anything! So water is actually the wisest choice: it hydrates you, providing the best environment physically and mentally for your body to function, and can reduce your 'sugar' cravings.

4) For lunch, which would you choose?

☐ **a) An egg-white omelette and some fresh fruit**

☐ **b) A fast-food takeaway**

☐ **c) A grilled chicken sandwich, packet of low-fat crisps and a banana**

Low-fat diets are popular for people trying to lose weight. Fat is the most calorie-dense food, so following a low-fat dies *will* help you cut calories, but it is not wise to starve yourself of good nutrition, which includes protein and essential fats. Egg-white omelettes and fruit may not give you all the calories and certainly not all the fat your body may need. General dietary advice is to reduce the overall amount of fat we are consuming. However, some fat, especially the good sources of fat, such as polyunsaturated and omega 3 fats found in nuts, seeds and oily fish, are essential for our health. Fast food – which can be very high in unhealthy saturated fat, refined sugars and refined carbohydrates – is a poor choice, best left for emergencies only. Sensible choices can be made: a chicken kebab with salad makes a great fast take-away, but leave out the hi-fat toppings and chilli sauces. A tasty sandwich, low-fat crisps and fruit will give your body all it needs to sustain you through the working day. Crisps may seem an unlikely health choice, but providing they are consumed in moderation, and eaten as part of a balanced meal (such as a lean chicken sandwich with watercress and thin slice of avocado plus a piece of fruit), this option would actually be your

healthiest. Substitute the bag of crisps with a bag of vegetable crudités and you've eaten one of the 5 recommended fruit and veg portions for the day. See page 224 for some menu ideas.

5) During the day, you:

☐ **a) Combat thirst when necessary by downing a lot of mineral water**

☐ **b) Limit yourself to 4 cups of tea and coffee, and then drink diet, caffeine-free sodas**

☐ **c) Sip water almost constantly, even when you don't feel thirsty**

By the time you feel thirsty, your body is already dehydrated. Sipping water throughout the day is a sensible tip, and will keep you well hydrated. Even your skin will benefit. Sipping little and often also provides the best opportunity for your body to hydrate itself effectively. Imagine your body as a house plant. If the plant gets dried up, it needs water, but if you watered it all at once with the amount of water it needs, the water would flood out of the bottom of the pot. Water the plant slowly throughout the day and you will find it absorbs what it needs and its healthy condition is fully restored. So think of that house plant, and drink little and often. Even though some sodas may be caffeine- and sugar-free, they don't add any nutritional value, and are better replaced by water.

6) What is your daily pattern?

- **a) Eat three substantial meals a day, and try to avoid snacking**
- **b) Eat less earlier in the day – because it's harder to resist naughty treats and snacks as the day wears on**
- **c) Eat 4 or 5 times a day – but keep the portion sizes smaller and well balanced**

A steady calorific intake spread evenly throughout the day can be a more successful eating strategy, especially if you suffer from lapses of energy. It is also important to eat the right balance of nutrients. For example, a little protein with some source of starch at lunchtime will aid concentration and energy levels through the afternoon. 'Starving-and-bingeing' is an unhealthy pattern to follow, and if you find that you're often tempted to snack later on in the day, focus on having some healthy snacks earlier together with some water to hydrate you. You may discover that the unhealthy sugar cravings that normally hit you will naturally reduce.

7) Before a visit to the gym, you:

- **a) Eat and drink lightly, to avoid exercising on a full stomach**
- **b) Eat a good lunch, to give your body plenty of energy**
- **c) Don't eat – save your appetite until afterwards**

Exercising on a full stomach is not a good idea and can be very uncomfortable. Your digestive system needs a supply of blood in order to digest food, but when you exercise your muscles also demand blood in order to carry oxen to the working muscles. This creates conflict as the body decides where the blood is most needed and can result in a stitch.

If you're planning to visit the gym, try to avoid eating for up to 2 hours beforehand, but do eat before this, as your body does need food to provide energy. However, it is advisable to start your training well hydrated. Drink a small cup of water about 30 minutes before you start training, and throughout your workout sip little and often – this will ensure that you have a more effective and enjoyable workout. See page 220 for more hydration hints.

8) After your workout, you:

- **a) Wait for half an hour, and then eat a light snack**
- **b) Eat a banana immediately to restore energy levels**
- **c) Take advantage of your revved-up metabolism and avoid eating, so you can burn off more fat**

Your muscle cells can replenish the essential glycogen stores most effectively within the first 2 hours after exercise. Foods such as bananas, dried fruits and wholegrain breads with natural fruit spreads are particularly good for this. But beware if you are training to lose weight. Eating too many of these foods after exercise can mean you have consumed more calories than you have just burnt off! A ripe banana, for instance, will give you a ready supply of simple sugars which can easily be converted into glycogen to help your body repair.

9) In the pub, what best describes your drinking and eating habits?

- **a) You choose 'long' drinks like wine spritzers or lagers, and avoid nibbling on crisps**
- **b) You drink whatever you like, but choose low-calorie mixers or colas to make up for the nuts you've munched**
- **c) You Drink wine or beer, but always have a glass of water in between each round.**

Alcohol is a diuretic, and while you're enjoying yourself at the pub your body will start feeling the effects of dehydration. By drinking water between each alcoholic drink, you'll not only help to combat the effects of dehydration, but be less likely to over-indulge on the alcohol front and minimize the chance of a bad head the following day. Nuts and crisps are high in fat and salt which will only increase your thirst. Too much salt can cause raised blood pressure. If you know that you have a heavy night's drinking ahead, it's a good idea to start the evening well hydrated. Make sure you have had your 2 litres/3$^{1}/_{2}$ of water before you start to party and hydrate as you go through the night. Drinking another 550ml/1 pint before your head hits the pillow, can also help minimize a sore head the next morning.

10) Last thing at night – what do you do?

☐ **a) Make sure you're full so you won't wake up hungry in the night**

☐ **b) Avoid eating at all – sleep on an empty stomach**

☐ **c) Eat some fresh fruit or raw vegetables, but make sure it's at least an hour before you go to sleep**

Some nutrition experts believe that eating too near bedtime can increase the chances of you storing the calories as fat – although going to bed hungry can lead to unsatisfying sleep patterns. If you are hungry and you have already eaten earlier in the evening, the best idea is to have a light fruit or vegetable snack, which will help stave off hunger pangs and, because it's low in fat and calories, it will not significantly add to your calorific intake, nor will it place heavy digestive demands on your body late at night. A glass of milk or a light carbohydrate snack such as small bowl of cereal can also be good, as they can stimulate feelings of calm through the release of specific brain transmitters.

How did you score?

Give yourself one point for every B answer, two points for every A answer, and 3 points for every C answer.

If you scored:

10–16 points

Your food IQ could use a good boost – and your body could well benefit from it too! It is not always easy to fit good nutrition into a busy life, so read on to find lots of advice to help you get the most out of your nutrition.

17–23 points

Your knowledge and food sense is pretty good, but the challenge often comes when you try to fit your knowledge into a busy life. So you should find all the tips here really helpful – and with prior planning, you'll benefit from more energy too.

24–30 points

You know your food facts, which means you are giving your body the best chance of an active and healthy life. Keep going, and the results will show for themselves.

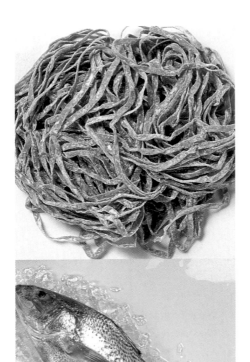

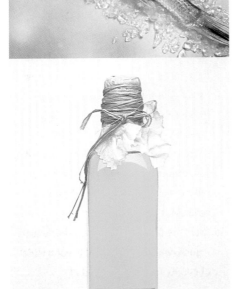

Calories and energy

All foods contain energy, which is measured in calorific units. The number of calories our bodies require depends on how active we are as well as the amount of muscle mass we have.

FOOD GROUP	CALORIES PER GRAM
Carbohydrates: Fruit, vegetables, starchy foods and sugars	4
Proteins: Meat, fish, pulses, dairy products	4
Fats: Oils, butter, lard, margarines	9

Most foods are composed of a variety of nutrients. However they tend to be classified according to their highest concentration: for example, potatoes are predominantly a starchy carbohydrate food but they also contain some protein and minute traces of fat. Nuts and seeds are considered proteins but also provide essential fats. Consequently the calorie values of different foods can vary widely within the groups and on cooking methods chosen. You can check some food values for yourself in the calorie tables on page 242.

The recommended daily calorie intake for a woman is 2,000, and 2,500 for a man.

What happens when we digest our food?

Enzymes along the digestive tract break down the food into smaller units that can be easily absorbed and used by the body. Carbohydrates break down to glucose molecules, fats to lipids and proteins to amino acids. These small micro-units then pass across the lining of the gut and into the bloodstream, where they are transported to the liver, the working muscles or fat cells. Glucose is our main source of energy, although we do break down fat from our fat cells as well. Glucose is stored in the muscle in the form of glycogen.

The amount of fuel our muscles use when we move our bodies depends on the intensity of the exercise. Muscle glycogen is the main fuel used for high-intensity effort, while fat contributes a greater proportion of energy in lower intensity exercise. When the supply of glycogen is depleted, the muscles' performance ability is significantly reduced. Consequently, long-duration high-intensity exercise such as endurance bike-riding and long hard running will be enhanced if you have more glycogen stored in the working muscles. What and when you eat can directly affect the amount of muscle glycogen your body can store. And it's not just your muscles that need fuel; your brain also needs a constant and steady supply.

Fresh, frozen or tinned?

Which do you choose? Although fresh organic fruit and vegetables are best, don't beat yourself up if you're not able to shop at your local farmers' market. Frozen and tinned sources can be a really useful addition to your shopping trolley. Supermarket fruit and vegetables can keep fresh a remarkably long time from the point of being picked, transported, stored in a warehouse and eventually ending up in your shopping trolley. While you're in the supermarket, stock up your store cupboard and freezer with tinned and frozen items. Studies have shown that the antioxidant content in tinned vegetables can be as high as fresh, and modern on-site food freezing techniques can actually mean frozen fruit and vegetables have a higher all-round nutrient content.

Bottom line? Do eat your minimum of 5 fruit and veg. servings a day and don't panic if they are not fresh. And remember, a glass of fruit or vegetable juice counts as a portion as well.

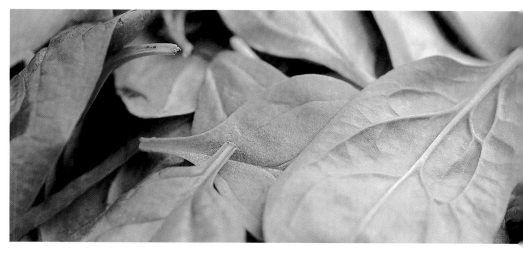

Good eating habits

1. Drink water, little and often, throughout the day.

2. Eat something in the morning – it does not have to be first thing as you jump out of bed, but eating something when you get up will replenish your blood glucose levels and fuel your brain and your body.

3. Eat at least 5 portions of fruit and vegetables a day – they're great as snacks if you have at least 1 serving per meal, you'll easily make this target.

4. Go for colour. Check you are eating a variety of colourful fruit and vegetables – think yellow, red, green and orange.

5. Eat as wide a variety of foods as possible. If you can count up the number of different foods you eat on your 10 fingers, you need to add more kinds to your diet. This will help you get a greater choice of nutrients and fibre sources.

6. Avoid long periods without eating. This will help stabilize your blood glucose levels and make you less likely to over-eat, or grab an unhealthy snack, later.

7. Rate your food hunger. On a scale of 1–5 (1 = starving, 5 = stuffed). Aim to eat before you reach '1' and stop eating before you reach '5'.

8. Take time to eat. It sounds obvious, but it will help you eat a more balanced diet and avoid excess calorie intake. Studies show that individuals eat up to 15% more calories when they are in a rush at meal times.

9. Chew your food. Proper chewing can aid your digestion, and has been shown to reduce symptoms of irritable bowel syndrome.

10. Avoid fad diets. There are no miracle foods – good health requires you to eat a variety of quality foods in moderation.

Major food groups

'Be wary' sources: Foods containing fat and sugar (9%)

Protein sources:

Milk and dairy products (12%)

Protein sources:

Meat, poultry, fish, eggs, beans, nuts and pulses (12%)

Carbohydrate sources:

Fruit and vegetables (33%)

Carbohydrate sources:

Bread, cereals, grains and potatoes (33%)

Foods containing fat and sugar

Butter, oil, margarine, cream cakes, chocolate, sweets, crisps and many drinks fall within this group. Many processed snack foods contain large amounts of fat, sugar and salt and so should be eaten occasionally and in small amounts. Choose low-fat spreads, low-sugar drinks and reduced-calorie mayonnaise and dips if you need to decrease your total calorie and fat intake. Processed foods can also be high in the damaging trans fats. These are usually listed on food labels as 'hydrogenated fats' and are best kept to a minimum in the diet.

Milk and dairy products

Calcium, a vital mineral for healthy bones, protein and important vitamins such as A, B12, D and riboflavin, are found in milk and dairy products. Enjoy them in moderation and try lower-fat options such as skimmed milk, low-fat yoghurts and reduced-fat cheeses. Children under 5 should be given full-fat milk and dairy products, as these contain essential nutrients for early growth. Children over 2 can, however, have semi-skimmed and those over 5 can have skimmed milk.

Meat, poultry, fish, eggs, beans, nuts and pulses

These are important elements of a healthy diet, as they contain protein, vitamins and minerals. Meat is a rich source of zinc, vitamin B12 and an easily absorbed form of iron. Some protein sources can be high in fats, so try lean cuts of meat or skinless chicken fillets. Fish oils contain omega 3 fatty acids, which are essential polyunsaturated fatty acids that reduce the risk of heart disease. It is recommended that portions of fish are eaten each week, one of which should be an oily variety such as salmon, tuna, mackerel, sardines, pilchards, herring or swordfish.

Fruit and vegetables

Eating more fruit and vegetables is one of the most important things we can do to improve our health and reduce the risk of heart disease, cancer and strokes. They also add colour, taste and texture to our food. Fruit and vegetables provide important amounts of vitamins C and A, folic acid and minerals such as iron, calcium and magnesium. They are naturally low in fat and sodium and provide a good amount of fibre. Choose a wide variety of types and colours each day to ensure you are getting a good balance. Dieticians and docters recommend a minimum of 5 portions of fruit and vegetables daily – fresh, frozen and juices all count.

Bread, cereals, grains and potatoes

These starchy foods are an important source of energy for the exercising body. Try to eat the wholegrain, brown or wholemeal varieties of bread and cereals to boost your intake of fibre, B vitamins, calcium and iron. And it's not just a plate of rice or pasta... this group also includes yams and plantains as well as sweet potatoes and wholegrain breakfast cereals.

Glycaemic index carbohydrates

Carbohydrate-rich foods are great energy suppliers for active people. When digested, carbohydrates break down into units of glucose, which enter the bloodstream and are then used by the body. Different sorts of carbohydrate foods, however, do not release glucose into the bloodstream at the same rate. Individual metabolic responses also influence the rate of absorption and digestion of nutrients, and these can have a direct impact on the quality of training, sports performance and recovery. The glycaemic index (GI) is a system of working out how quickly carbohydrates are broken down and digested, and how effectively they raise your blood sugar levels. An increase in the blood glucose level, will stimulate insulin production (insulin is produced in the pancreas, to to normalize/reduce blood sugar levels).

The GI rates range from 1 to 100 (100 is glucose). Anything below 55 is considered to be low, 55–85 is medium and anything above 85 is high. High GI foods are those that provide a fast release of glucose into the bloodstream, medium GI foods a moderate release, and low GI foods provide a more gradual release.

GI foods for energy and activity

(1) After a hard exercise class or training session, consume more carbohydrate foods with a high GI, preferably within 2 hours. This will boost the muscles' ability to replenish depleted muscle glycogen. However, total daily carbohydrate intake is still important to aid muscle glucose replenishment.

(2) At the start of the day, you may find it suits you best to consume more moderate to low GI carbohydrates. This will provide you with a slow release of energy and sustain your energy levels. Some individuals find a low to moderate GI breakfast such as a bowl of porridge with some fruit a very effective way to tackle mid-morning hunger pangs.

The concept of GI carbohydrates is fairly new. Refer to the tables on pages 245–7 to help you assess the GI of the foods you eat. If you are susceptible to energy swings you may find this approach particularly useful.

Vitamins and minerals

Vitamins and minerals are important for our immune system and daily health. A balanced diet of fruit, vegetables, meat, fish and wholegrains provides us with all the vitamins and minerals we need.

However, the stresses of daily life, increased consumption of processed foods and incidence of food health scares have created an environment in which more of us are reaching for the supplement bottle. While an adequate supply of vitamins and minerals is essential to our health, certain nutrients can be dangerous and lead to irreversible health problems if dosage is excessive. There are guidelines that advise you of the safe limits. More is not necessarily better and you can get too much of a good thing! Have a look at the table on page 248–9.

RDA

'RDA' stands for 'recommended dietary allowance'. The RDA is the intake that meets the nutrient needs of a healthy person. Recent research has indicated that the RDA levels represent the minimum intake, and consequently revised recommendations have now suggested upper tolerable intake limits (UL).

UL

The UL is the highest vitamin or mineral dose that can be taken without risk of adverse effects. This is not a recommended level of intake, since there does not appear to be any additional health benefits at intake levels above the RDA.

Sports nutrition

Nutritional guidelines for sports men and women aim to provide the training body with the appropriate amount of fluid and fuel to match their energy demands, help control body temperature and hydration status. The general advice for high intensity sports, such as hockey, tennis, badminton and soccer, and paced steady-state sports, such as endurance running, hiking and cycling, is to consume a diet high in complex carbohydrates complemented by a moderate intake of protein and essential fat is also recommended.

If you are a serious athlete, you need a foundation of carbohydrates in each meal to fuel your muscles. Some protein is important to build, protect and maintain muscles, but too much can displace carbohydrate. Athletes should aim for a 3–5g intake of carbohydrate per 450g/1lb of body weight. You will find the GI chart useful to help you calculate your carbohydrate needs (see pages 245–7).

Nutrional guidelines for athletes

1. **Between 60 and 70% of your calorific intake should be from carbohydrates.**
2. **Drink 220–440ml/8–16fl oz of a rapidly absorbed fluid (water or sports drink)** 10–15 minutes before exercise, and at least 110–275ml/4–10fl oz every 15–20 minutes during exercise.
3. **Make sure you get enough calories. Monitor your diet to check that you have an adequate intake of vitamins, minerals and proteins.**

Female athletes should also:

1. **Consume 800–1,200mg of calcium daily. Amenorrhoeic athletes (those whose mensruation has stopped) should consume 1,500mg daily.**
2. **Consider increasing your iron intake, particularly from animal sources, which can be absorbed more efficiently than from vegetable sources. If there is a history of ammenorrhoea, it is advisable to get your GP to monitor your iron status regularly with blood tests and dietary iron intake. The recommended daily intake is 15mg. See the vitamin and mineral table for iron sources (see pages 248–9).**

Pre-workout nutrition

Any serious exerciser who is concerned about getting the most from their workout wants to know what is best to eat beforehand. Preferences vary from person to person, and according to the type of exercise. Before high-impact activities such as running, you need to think more carefully about what to eat than you would before exercise during which the stomach remains a little more stable, like cycling.

Most of us lead busy lives that have us rushing from work to fit in our

Top tips:

We are all different – so to determine the right pre-training fuel for you, experiment using the guidelines below. These are only guidelines, and preferences will vary according to time of day, type of workout and level of intensity.

- **Avoid sugary foods.**
- **Avoid food that is too bulky or has too high a fibre content, as you will be more prone to abdominal discomfort.**
- **Allow adequate time for food to digest. The general rule is 3–4 hours for a large meal, 2–3 hours for a smaller meal, 1–2 hours for a blended or liquid meal, and less than an hour for a snack, depending on your own tolerance. Allow more time to digest your food before intense exercise.**
- **Eat foods that contain some carbohydrate but are low in fat, protein and fibre.**
- **Select foods that are easy to digest, such as those listed in Snacking on the Run, page 218.**
- **And always have a drink as well, so that as you are addressing your blood glucose levels, you're also hydrating your body.**

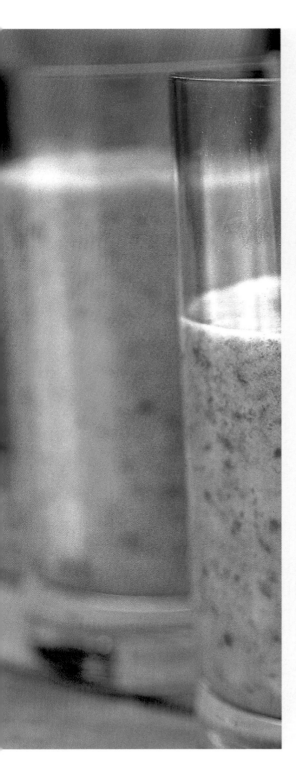

Snacking on the run

Each of these snacks is around 300 calories.

Raspberry Smoothie

Mix 2 cups low-fat fortified soy milk, 1 cup frozen raspberries (no added sugar), ½ banana, ¼ cup light tofu, and 1 teaspoon sugar (or to taste) in a blender.

Peanut Toast

2 slices of wholegrain toast spread with 2 teaspoons peanut butter and 1 small sliced banana.

Cinnamon and Apple Bagel

Mix chopped ½ apple with 1 tablespoon fat-free cream cheese and ¼ teaspoon ground cinnamon. Spread on ½ wholewheat bagel.
Accompaniment: small glass of orange juice.

Trail Mix

Combine 2 teaspoons dried cranberries, 2 tablespoons raisins, and 2 tablespoons peanuts.
Accompaniment: small glass of skimmed milk.

Wholewheat Cereal

35g/1¼oz wholeweat flaked breakfast cereal with skimmed milk.

workouts. With such tight schedules, care with nutrition can often take a back seat, not only through lack of time but also lack of pre-planning. However, keeping mindful of a few facts can help. Studies have shown, for example, that taking a small amount (approximately 50g/2oz) of carbohydrate (in solid or liquid form) just before exercise can help maintain blood glucose levels, delay fatigue and improve performance.

Pre-exercise nutrition should:

1. **Help establish optimum blood glucose levels necessary for muscle uptake.**
2. **Halt a grumbling stomach.**
3. **Fuel muscles for the workout: appropriate food eaten far enough in advance can be digested and refuel muscle glycogen levels.**
4. **Increase mental performance through confidence that the body is well fuelled for the work ahead.**

Hydration

Most of us know we need to stay well hydrated to keep the body functioning efficiently. A 2-litre/3½-pint fluid intake per day is often cited as the recommended amount for people who are not exercising. This fluid can be made up from water-based fruit and vegetables as well as more liquid foods such as soups. Recent evidence suggests it is also important to keep well hydrated to avoid the risk of kidney stones and some bowel cancers. Consuming just 6 glasses of water a day as opposed to the recommended 8 glasses a day could put you at risk. In addition, stress, air-conditioned environments, heat and frequent cups of caffeinated beverages such as coffee, tea and soda drinks all contribute to dehydration.

When we exercise, hydration becomes even more crucial. Drinking replenishes vital fluids and electrolytes (such as sodium and potassium), cools the body and can provide a source of energy to refuel depleting muscle glycogen levels. Most fitness enthusiasts believe that dehydration occurs only in extreme situations, but when you are working out, it can happen any time someone loses fluid and does not replace it. Inadequate fluid intake causes dehydration, which directly reduces performance and contributes to heat illness.

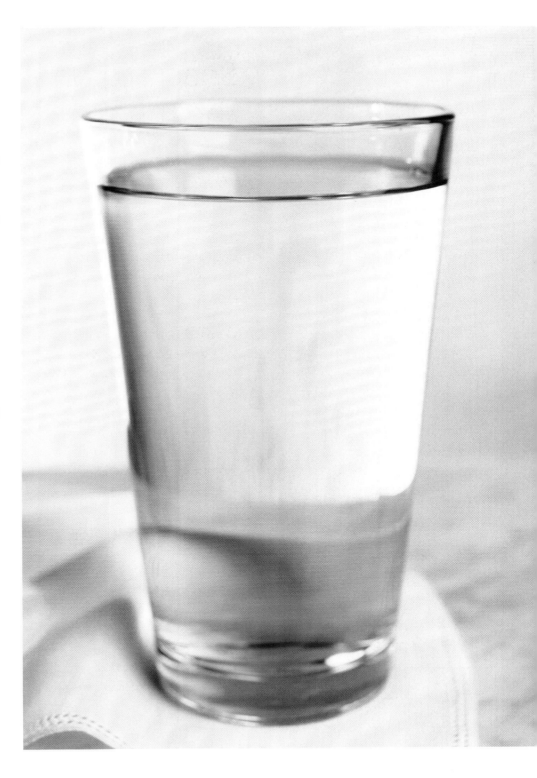

Hydration hints

Take a gulp.

Gauge the amount of fluid you consume by gulps, as one gulp usually equals about 2.75ml/1fl oz.

Drink to schedule, not by thirst.

By the time you become thirsty you may already be dehydrated. Schedule in breaks for drinking before, during and after activity workouts.

Know the warning signs.

If you are not used to keeping yourself well hydrated, your thirst mechanism may well be suppressed and you will be unable to detect the warning signs until it is too late. Light-headedness, headaches, dark urine, dry mouth and lips are all signs of dehydration. To re-educate your thirst mechanism, try to drink 8 glasses of water spread throughout the day for 3 weeks. Slowly you will find that the hypothalamus message centre in your brain will tell you when you are thirsty again.

Water through your day

Make hydration part of your lifestyle by always having healthy fluids on hand and taking time for fluid breaks. Here are some hints:

- Have a glass of diluted fruit juice first thing in the morning and aim to consume 4 glasses of water by the end of lunchtime. This way you will not be playing catch-up for the rest of the day.
- Place 8 pebbles into a small bowl, and every time you have a glass of water transfer one of the pebbles into an empty bowl. By the end of the day, aim to have transferred all the pebbles from one bowl to the other.
- Carry a water bottle with you. If you spend a lot of time in the car, carry a pull-top bottle, which you can drink when the car is stationary.
- Encourage your children to drink only water or diluted fruit juice. If they do have soft drinks, limit the amount – try to restrict them to one meal a day.
- Keep a water bottle by your lavatory. As strange as this may sound, it can prompt you to drink water and replace the fluids you have lost.

How much should I drink?

The more active you are the more fluid you should consume.

Less active: 8–10 glasses a day. This is the equivalent of 1.8–2.2 litre/64–78fl oz.

More active: drink at least 10–12 glasses per day. This is the equivalent of 2.2–2.6 litres/78–92fl oz.

Experts recommend that when you exercise you should drink at least 440ml/16fl oz before you start.

110–220ml/4–8fl oz every 15–20 minutes during strenuous exercise. Post-exercise, replenish with 660ml/24fl oz.

Water facts

1. **Research shows that exercisers tend to replenish only 50% of the fluid lost during a typical workout.**
2. **As little as 2% dehydration can cause cardiovascular endurance to fall by 6–7%.**
3. **Exercisers who begin a workout well hydrated and maintain their hydration throughout may last 33% longer those who don't drink anything.**
4. **Dehydration can make the exercise session feel harder. This is particularly a problem if you are new to exercise, as your body will be experiencing a new sensation that may not be that comfortable. Going into your workout dehydrated will only make your new decision to become fit more questionable!**
5. **Taste preferences can change with exercise, and some flavours can encourage increased fluid uptake. This can be particularly important in children who do not have a well-developed thirst mechanism and can be more prone to heat exhaustion. Orange- and grape-flavoured drinks have been shown to be the biggest thirst stimulators for children.**
6. **If you are a Java junkie, avoid using caffeinated beverages (such as colas) as a way of hydrating, as they can inhibit effective rehydration by increasing fluid loss as urine.**

What should I drink – water or a sports drink?

During exercise a sports drink is better, but in a long-distance endurance event such as a marathon, runners usually choose to alternate between water and sports drinks at the drinking stations. Not all sports drinks are created equal. Here's what to look for:

Carbohydrates:

Why? Important for replenishing lost muscle fuel in the form of muscle glycogen. While it will be difficult to replenish all your muscle glycogen while exercising, the sugars will boost essential blood glucose. Look for a mix of glucose, sucrose and fructose on the label – but check that fructose is the least amount, as drinking large quantities can cause abdominal pain.

Calories:

Some sports drinks are designed for serious athletes requiring significant energy replenishment, providing 50–60 calories per 220ml/8fl oz. If you want to lose weight, be wary not to choose a sports drink high in calories, or better still, make your own (see right).

Electrolytes:

When we sweat we lose essential electrolytes such as sodium and potassium. These minerals encourage drinking and help to restore fluid balance. At least 100mg of sodium and 28mg of potassium per 220ml/8 fl oz is recommended.

Avoid carbonation:

Fizzy bubbles can make it difficult to drink quickly during exercise and make you feel full, limiting the overall amount of fluid you drink.

Staying hydrated is important for us all when exercising, but it is especially important for pregnant women and children, as they are particularly prone to overheating. Children often don't notice when this is happening as their bodies' thermoregulation system is not fully developed.

A word about coffee

If you love coffee, don't panic! – you don't need to give up your mug of Java. Caffeine has been shown to stimulate brain function and can also play a useful part in the exercise process. Drinking a cup of black unsweetened coffee or green tea before you exercise can enhance performance. Coffee stimulates the release of fatty acids into the bloodstream, which can be used as a source of fuel during cardiovascular exercise. Just remember to allow 30 minutes between drinking your beverage and doing your exercise. Oh, and you do need to do the exercise to burn off those fats in your bloodstream – drinking your coffee and then sitting still reading the papers, sadly, will not have the same effect!

Make your own sports drink

You can make your own sports drink to help replenish lost minerals and electrolytes and restore your energy levels. The addition of a little salt is important because it aids the absorption of electrolytes across the stomach wall.

110ml/4fl oz orange juice
440ml/16fl oz water
Pinch of salt

Dissolve the salt in a little warm water. Add the orange juice and cold water. Shake well. Keep your drink at room temperature. Fluids that are too cold exit the stomach quickly, before the essential minerals and glucose have been absorbed.

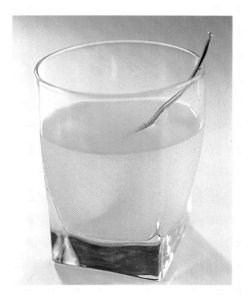

Menu ideas

We all lead busy lives and squeezing in exercise can be a problem. When you are unsure about what to eat to optimize your training as well, life becomes doubly confusing, so have a look at these sample menus as they may help you to put together menu plans to suit the activity in which you are involved.

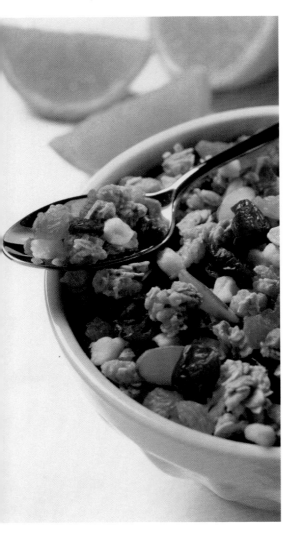

Case Study

Cathy is a PA who works long hours at her desk. She attends an aerobics class twice a week and goes hiking at the weekends.

Cathy's job is predominantly sedentary, and she would describe herself as moderately active. Her calorie requirements are between 1,800 and 2,200. She lives alone and often gets home late after going to the gym. She does not like red meat but enjoys fish. Since Cathy's office is air-conditioned and her job quite stressful, it is especially important that she consumes 2 litres/3½ pints of water throughout the day – so she opts out of the office coffee and gets water instead. She needs meal ideas that are quick and easy to prepare and cook.

Sample menu plan

On waking:
Glass of water.

Breakfast:
Toasted English muffin with 2 teaspoons peanut butter topped with 1 sliced plum.
Cup of coffee or tea and a glass of water.

Lunch:
Jacket potato with tuna, chopped tomatoes and peppers.
200ml/7fl oz glass orange juice.

Pre-workout snack:
Shop-bought fruit smoothie and 1 small banana.

[Aerobics class]

Supper:
Mediterranean Pasta
Heat 1 cup frozen broccoli spears, ½ cup tinned white kidney beans and ½ cup favourite vegetable-based pasta sauce in a microwave-able dish for about 3 minutes, or until heated through. Serve over 1 cup cooked pasta.
Low-fat natural yoghurt.

Case Study

Sarah is a weekend warrior. She was very sporty at college but since having a family as well as a job working from home, she gets her physical kicks from local competitive events. She manages to train 3 times during the week and likes to do an event once a month, whether it's a 5km/3.1 mile run for her daughter's school or the London to Brighton bike ride. Sarah needs, depending on her training, 2,100–2,500 calories a day.

Sample menu plan

On waking:
Hot oatmeal porridge made with semi-skimmed milk topped with blueberries and a sprinkle of wheatgerm. 1 slice wholemeal toast with marmite

[45-minute cardio-interval session]

Lunch:
Small bowl of cooked pasta with home-made tomato sauce and a feta cheese side salad.

Snack:
Small handful of nuts.
Small glass of orange juice.

Supper:
Chicken with Couscous (see page 227) with spinach and sweet potato.
Cantaloupe melon and kiwi fruit salad with natural yoghurt.

Case Study

Peter, a management accountant, is a 70kg/154lb tri-athlete who trains twice a day. As an ex-professional athlete, he is well aware of the energy demands he places on his body. His daily calorie requirements are 3,000–3,300.

Sample menu plan

On waking:
Glass of diluted fruit juice.
[Resistance training session]

Breakfast:
Large bowl of wholewheat cereal with 300ml/11fl oz semi-skimmed milk

Snack:
Tuna sandwich (2 slices bread).
2 pieces fruit.

Lunch:
2 jacket potatoes with 225g/8oz baked beans and a side salad.
Glass of tomato juice.
Piece of fruit and yoghurt.

Snack:
Wholegrain crackers with peanut butter.
Small banana.
[Cardiovascular training session]

Supper:
175g/6oz cooked pasta with tomato and vegetable sauce and 150g/5oz chicken breast, dark green leafy vegetables, 1 cob sweetcorn.
Small bowl of ice cream.
Glass of orange juice.

Snack:
2 slices toast with natural fruit jam spread topped with sliced banana.

Recipes

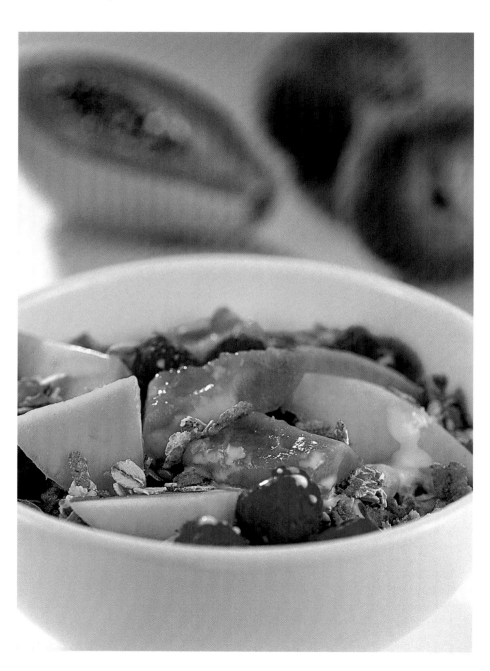

Breakfast ideas

Porridge with Forest Fruits

Serves 1

Calories: 411

Carbohydrate: 68.6g

Fat: 6.1g

Protein: 22g

Cook ½ cup porridge oats with 1 cup skimmed milk and 1 cup water. Add fresh strawberries and blueberries just before serving.

Wholewheat Breakfast Cereal

Serves 1

Calories: 458

Carbohydrate: 87.4g

Fat: 8.5g

Protein: 10.8g

Mix 1 cup cooked bulgur wheat with 2 teaspoons brown sugar, 2 tablespoons chopped dried apricots and 1 tablespoon chopped walnuts. Serve with semi-skimmed milk.

English Muffins with Cream Cheese and Plums

Serves 1

Calories: 167

Carbohydrate: 29g

Fat: 1.3g

Protein: 9.4g

Toast an English muffin. Spread a thin layer of low-fat cream cheese on each slice, top with sliced plum and sprinkle with nutmeg.

Toast and Eggs

Serves 1
Calories 326
Carbohydrate 48.5g
Fat 9g
Protein 16g
Toast 2 slices wholegrain bread and serve with a poached egg and 2 grilled tomatoes.

Breakfast in a Bottle

Serves 1
Calories: 218
Carbohydrate: 37.3g
Fat: 2.1g
Protein: 15.1g
Blend together ½ small tub low-fat plain yoghurt, a handful of wholewheat breakfast flakes, 1 small can de-stoned prunes in natural juice, 275ml/10fl oz soya or skimmed milk and 4 ice cubes. Blend and go.

Lunches

Turkey Salad Sandwich

Spicy turkey salad with sweet peppers, corn and green onions. Colourful, crunchy and packed with vitamins.
Makes: 4 sandwiches
Calories: 280

Carbohydrate: 40g
Fat: 3g
Protein: 24g

200g/7oz cooked turkey or chicken
1 small sweet pepper, finely chopped
2 tablespoons tinned sweetcorn
2 spring onions, finely chopped
2 tablespoons plain low-fat yoghurt
Handful of fresh basil, chopped
Pinch of ground cumin
Pinch of salt
8 slices multi-grain bread

In a bowl combine the turkey, pepper, corn, spring onions, yoghurt, basil, cumin and salt. Make 4 sandwiches using equal amounts of turkey salad. Serve with a handful of carrot sticks.

Salmon Niçoise Pittas

Red-leaf lettuce is low-calorie, high in fibre and a good source of vitamin A.
Serves 2
Calories: 362
Carbohydrate: 34g
Fat: 5g
Protein: 32g

150g/5oz tinned salmon, skinless and boneless
90g/3¾oz green beans, cooked
2 plum tomatoes
4 black olives, pitted and finely chopped
2 tablespoons finely chopped red onion

2 tablespoons snipped fresh dill
1 teaspoon olive oil
2 tablespoons lemon juice
Pinch of black pepper
2 wholewheat pitta bread rounds
Fresh young spinach

Mix the salmon, green beans, tomatoes, olives, onion, dill, oil, lemon juice and pepper together in a large bowl. Line the pitta breads with several spinach leaves, then fill with the salmon mixture.

Quick Chinese Savoury Rice

Use up lean cooked meat or any leftovers from your fridge to make this quick and nutritious meal.
Serves 4
Calories: 255
Carbohydrate: 38g
Fat: 5g
Protein: 17g

1 small onion, chopped
4 tablespoons chopped green pepper
150g/5oz sugar snap peas
1 tablespoon canola or olive oil
165g/5½oz cups cooked rice
150g/5oz drained chopped water chestnuts
150g/5oz chopped mushrooms
4 tablespoons reduced-salt soy sauce
175g/6oz of cooked chicken, prawns or lean meat
150g/5oz beansprouts
2 egg whites

In a wok, cook and stir the onion, green pepper and sugar-snap peas in a little oil until the onion is tender. Stir in the rice, water chestnuts, mushrooms and soy sauce. Cook over a low heat for 10 minutes, stirring to avoid sticking.

Add the meat, or prawns, and beansprouts and heat through. Just before serving, add the egg whites and stir until the egg starts to set.

Chicken Tortilla Wraps

Enjoy these wraps, rich in vitamin E and essential protein. Dip them into spicy salsa for a kick to your lunch!

Serves 4

Calories: 310

Carbohydrate: 37g

Fat: 8g

Protein: 26g

4 flour tortillas, 18cm/7in across

2 cooked chicken breasts, chopped

1 tablespoon grated low-fat hard cheese

1 small red onion, finely chopped

1 yellow pepper, finely sliced

1 crushed clove garlic

1 teaspoon ground cumin

1 small ripe avocado, sliced

1 small bag of watercress, washed

Chopped parsley, to garnish

Combine the chicken, cheese, onion, pepper, garlic and cumin in a bowl. Spread an equal amount of the mixture on each tortilla, add the sliced avocado and a handful of watercress. Garnish with the chopped parsley and serve with cherry tomatoes or a side salad.

Red pepper and tomato soup with orange

Rich in antioxidants, this soup is a great immune booster. It freezes well, and is great after long, cold walks in the winter.

Serves 8

Calories: 117

Carbohydrate: 20g

Fat: 4g

Protein: 2.5g

4 teaspoons olive oil

2 carrots, chopped

2 medium onions, chopped

4 crushed garlic cloves

2 red peppers, seeds discarded and chopped

Pinch of allspice

1 tablespoon tomato purée

3 x 400g/14oz tins tomatoes in rich tomato sauce

1 chicken or vegetable stock cube

375ml/14fl oz water

450ml/16fl oz fresh orange juice

Large handful of chopped basil

Salt and pepper

Heat the oil in a pan, add the carrots and onions and cook gently for 5 minutes. Add garlic, red peppers and ground allspice and cook for a further 3–4 minutes.

Mix in the tomato purée, tomatoes, stock cube and water and simmer for 10–15 minutes until the vegetables are tender. Take off the heat, then add the orange juice and chopped basil. Season well.

Serve with wholemeal mixed grain roll and low-fat cream cheese.

Dinners

Low-fat Spinach Lasagne

A great-tasting meatless alternative to traditional lasagne

Serves 4

Calories: 230

Carbohydrate: 27g

Fat: 6g

Protein: 16g

2 tablespoons tomato purée

1 tablespoon Italian seasoning

Pinch of chilli powder

Salt and pepper

400g/14oz whole tomatoes

2 tablespoons grated low-fat Cheddar cheese

2 tablespoons grated mozzarella cheese

2 tablespoons low-fat cottage cheese

450g/1lb cooked lasagne pasta sheets

450g/1lb cooked spinach

To make the sauce, combine the tomato purée, Italian seasoning, chilli powder, salt and pepper with the juice from the tinned tomatoes. Mix in the cheeses, saving some grated cheese for the top.

Place enough sauce mixture on the bottom of a lasagne dish to cover. Add a layer of the lasagne sheets, then a layer of spinach, then a layer of sauce. Add another layer of lasagne, then a layer of whole tomatoes. Add thec heeses and the remainder of the sauce and sprinkle with the reserved grated cheese.

Bake for 45 minutes–1 hour at 180°C/350°F/gas mark 4. Be sure to let the lasagne set for 15 minutes before serving. Serve with a mixed green salad.

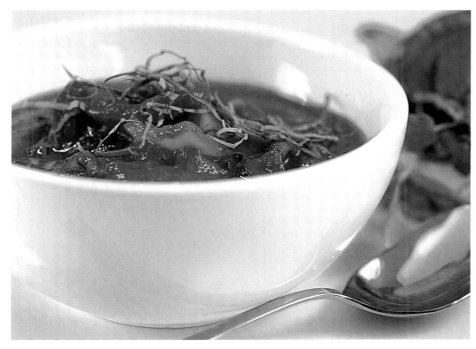

Red Pepper and Tomato Soup with Orange

Warm Fennel and Cannellini Bean Salad

Serves 2

Calories: 297

Carbohydrate: 49g

Fat: 2g

Protein: 17g

150g/5oz fresh fennel bulb

150g/5oz courgette

100g/4oz green pepper

150ml/5fl oz white wine

6 pitted green olives, sliced

2 tablespoon fresh mint leaves

Salt and pepper

800g/1³⁄₄lb canned cannellini or other white beans

30g/1oz rocket or baby spinach leaves

Finely dice the fennel, courgette and green pepper. Place in a large saucepan with the white wine, olives, ¹⁄₂ tablespoon of the mint leaves and some salt and pepper. Bring to the boil and simmer for 5 minutes or until the vegetables are tender.

Rinse and drain the canned beans. When the vegetables are soft, add them to the pan and heat through for 5 minutes. Just before serving, stir through the rocket or baby spinach leaves and season to taste with salt and pepper. Serve garnished with the remaining mint leaves cut into fine shreds. Serve with mixed wild rice.

Chicken with Coucous

Coucous is small grains of semolina pasta. It's a rich source of low GI carbohydrates and makes a great side dish with chicken or other cooked meats.

Serves 6

Calories: 328

Carbohydrate: 22g

Fat: 16g

Protein: 23g

1¹⁄₂ teaspoons ground cumin

¹⁄₂ teaspoon ground cinnamon

Pinch of salt

Pinch of cayenne pepper

6 x 120g/4¹⁄₂oz skinless, boneless chicken thighs

2 medium sweet potatoes, peeled and cut into
  2.5cm/1 in cubes

3 cloves garlic, crushed

550ml/1 pint water

100g/4oz frozen peas

175g/6oz coucous

2 tablespoons lemon juice

Chopped fresh mint, to garnish.

Heat the oven to 190°C/375°F/gas mark 5. Combine the cumin, cinnamon, salt and cayenne pepper in a small bowl and mix well.

Trim the fat from the chicken thighs, rub on some spice mixture and leave to one side. Reserve the remaining spice mixture.

In a medium flameproof casserole dish, combine the sweet potatoes, garlic and remaining spice mixture. Mix well, top with the chicken and add enough water to cover. Bring to the boil, add the peas, cover and place in the oven. Bake for about 25 minutes until the chicken is cooked through and the sweet potatoes are tender.

Remove the casserole from the oven. Sprinkle the coucous on top, pushing it into the liquid with a spoon. Cover and let stand until the liquid is absorbed (about 5–10 minutes). Drizzle with lemon juice, garnish with mint and serve immediately. Serve with roasted tomatoes and peppers.

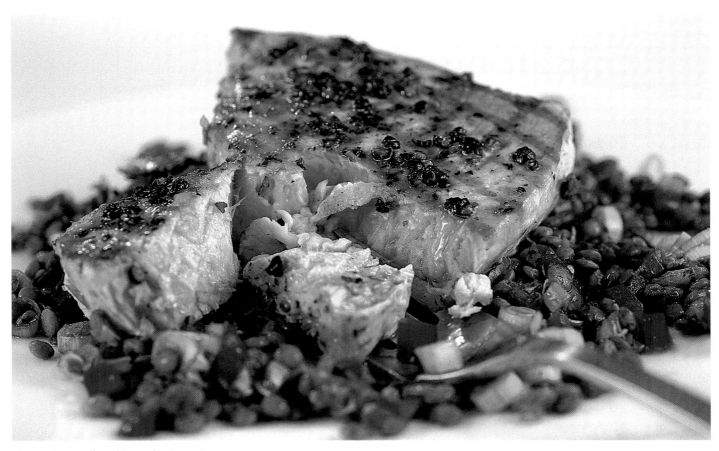

Peppered Swordfish with Lentil Taboulleh

Peppered Swordfish with Lentil Taboulleh

Serves 2

Calories: 838

Carbohydrate: 68g

Fat: 37g

Protein: 60.8g

2 thick, meaty pieces swordfish, or tuna if you prefer

Rock salt and cracked pepper

1–2 tablespoons light olive oil

250g/8oz puy lentils, or continental green lentils

1 small onion, peeled

1 clove garlic

1 red pepper

1 shallot

2 spring onions

Large handful of chopped fresh coriander and flat leaf parsley

1 tablespoon balsamic vinegar

3–4 tablespoons extra virgin olive oil

Extra generous grinding of salt and pepper

Trim the fish of any dark flesh or skin. Season lightly with rock salt and then evenly coat each steak with the cracked black pepper, pressing it firmly into the fish. This can be done up to 48 hours before cooking.

To cook the lentils, first rinse them well 2–3 times under cold water. Put into a saucepan with double the volume of cold water. Add the onion whole, and the clove of garlic. Bring the water to the boil and simmer with a lid on for 15 minutes for the puy lentils or 20–25 minutes for the continental green variety. Never season the lentils before they are cooked, or they will be tough. When they are just *'al dente'* drain them well, discarding the onion and garlic.

Meanwhile, deseed the red pepper and chop very finely, along with the shallot and the spring onions. Add to the hot drained lentils, along with the chopped herbs. Put in the balsamic vinegar and olive oil and season very well. Pulses in general do need a lot of seasoning. Whilst the lentils are cooling down, heat a heavy frying pan until it is smoking. Sear the fish for 1 minute on each side. Serve immediately on a bed of the lentils.

The lentil mixture can be kept for up to 3 days and is equally good cold. Serve with a spinach salad with tomatoes, asparagus, avocado and yellow peppers.

Gammon Steaks with Thai-style Salsa

Quick and easy to prepare. This dish gives you a supper rich in antioxidants, iron and zinc.

Serves 2

Calories: 347

Carbohydrate: 28g

Fat: 14g

Protein: 30g

2 gammon steaks
vegetable oil spray

For the salsa:
100g/4oz tomatoes
100g/4oz cucumber
100g/4oz carrots
50g/2oz celery
50g/2oz spring onions
1 tablespoon chopped fresh coriander
6 tablespoons lime or lemon juice
1–2 teaspoons fish sauce or soy sauce, to taste
4 tablespoons mild sweet chilli sauce

First make the salsa. Chop all the vegetables very finely and place in a bowl. Stir in the remaining ingredients and set aside to marinate while you cook the gammon.

Heat a griddle or heavy-based frying pan over a very high heat. Spritz the pan with vegetable oil spray, then lay the gammon steaks in the pan and lower the heat to medium. Cook for about 3 minutes on each side, or until nicely browned and hot. Serve with the salsa and steamed wild rice.

Liquid refreshment

Smoothies and juices can be a great way to increase your nutrient intake. They can make easy hydrating energy boosters or supplement breakfasts on the go. Here are just a few ideas:

Apple, Carrot and Ginger

Juice of 2 apples, 3 carrots and 2.5cm/1in cube of peeled, fresh ginger.

Fennel, Cucumber, Mint and Apple

1 fennel bulb, 15cm/6in cucumber, large handful of mint leaves and 3 apples.

Antioxidant Super Booster

275ml/10fl oz soya milk or skimmed milk, a handful of blueberries, strawberries, ½ banana, 1 tablespoon wheatgerm, and 4 ice cubes.

Healthy Chocolate Indulgence

275ml/10fl oz skimmed milk, 1 sachet low-fat instant hot chocolate drink dissolved in a little hot water, pinch of freshly grated nutmeg, ½ frozen peeled banana, 1 tablespoon wheatgerm and 4 ice cubes.

Hot Lemon and Ginseng Wake-up Call

This is a great substitute for caffeine and provides excellent immune-boosting health properties as well.

Hot water with juice of 1 lemon, ½ teaspoon honey, 1 tablespoon fresh liquid ginseng (from health-food shops).

NB! Gingseng is not suitable for everyone. If you are hypertensive (have high blood pressure), please avoid.

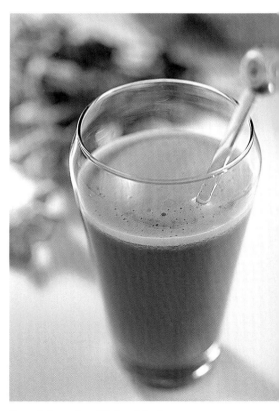

Fennel, Cucumber, Mint and Apple

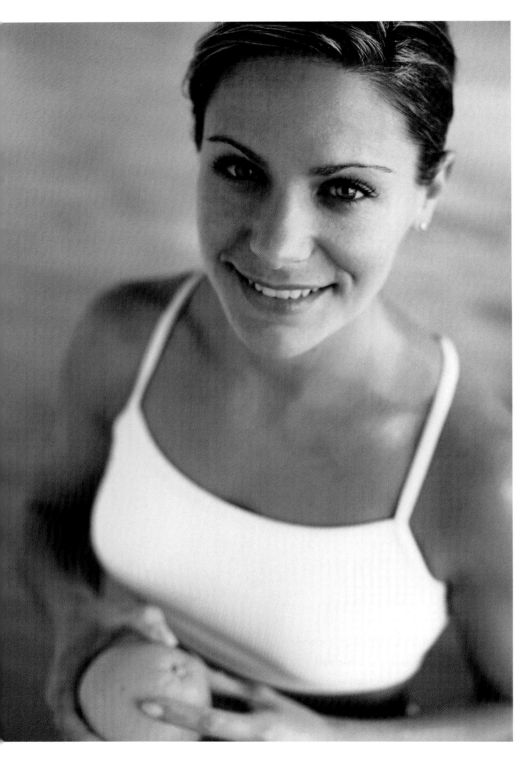

Questions and Answers

Q I am a tri-athlete and I eat very little protein. I'm concerned that I should be supplementing my diet with protein powder. However, the protein shakes I see in the shops seem very expensive and confusing. How can I make my own?

A Packaged protein powders and shakes are expensive. You can easily make your own version for less than 2p/3c per gram of protein. Here is a quick and simple recipe for a high-protein drink.

In a blender, mix 1 cup skimmed milk, 2 tablespoons skimmed milk powder, 2 tablespoons instant pudding mix (this thickens the shake to a more satisfying consistency; pick your favourite flavour) and add 4 ice cubes. Blend for until the ice cubes have disappeared. Add a few frozen banana chunks and berries to taste, as these will also boost the antioxidant capacity of the shake. This drink provides around 16 grams of protein. Also think about adding natural sources of protein to your meals. Tinned tuna and cottage cheese will boost your protein needs without you having to cook or stretch your budget too much.

Q I am an aerobics enthusiast participating in 3–4 exercise classes a week. What is the recommended amount of protein, carbohydrates and fat that I would need to sustain weight and increase energy levels?

A In order to sustain weight, an individual has to eat sufficient calories to match their total energy output. This is highly individual and depends on many factors such as body size, age, gender and fitness level. Very roughly speaking, let's say that an athletic female participant would require 2,500 calories per day. The carbohydrate group should supply 50–55% of calories, from as many unrefined sources as possible. Fats including fish, seed and grain oils should supply 20–25%. The remaining calories should come from the protein group. Also, don't forget vitamins and minerals taken from a broad range of vegetable and fruit groups. You should aim for a minimum 5 portions per day, predominantly from vegetable sources.

Q I really like fizzy cola. Can I use this as a good rehydration drink?

A Diet soda drinks do not make good sports drink as they do not contain any carbohydrate for replenishing lost glucose, nor do they provide enough sodium or potassium optimally to replenish these lost electrolytes. Regular soda drinks can have a high fructose content which, coupled with their carbonation, can lead to abdominal pain during exercise.

Q I've switched to a vegetarian diet to help me lose weight, but I still don't seem to be losing any weight. Why?

A When you are trying to lose weight the total number of calories as well as the nutrients consumed is important. Your calorie intake will depend on your body size and level of activity. Generally speaking, to lose 450g/1lb of weight a week you need to expend an additional 3,500 calories over the course of a week. Switching to a balanced vegetarian diet is an important health decision but it does not necessarily guarantee you a decrease in calorific intake. Indeed as a vegetarian you may well be consuming more calories through an increased consumption of cheese and nuts. Cheese, while undoubtedly a good source of calcium, can be high in calories and saturated fat. A 50g/2oz cube of Cheddar will provide you with roughly 17g/¹/₂oz of fat! Focus on fruit and vegetables as well as pulses, with wholegrains to help keep your diet balanced, and this way you will avoid saturated fat. In addition, do watch your portion size. You may find a dietary analysis programme of use, to help you work out a balanced diet.

Q I work all day in a office and go straight to the gym on my way home, but I often find I get light-headed when I work out. What should I do?

A If you are feeling light-headed, it may well be because you are exercising too intensively too quickly, reducing bloodflow to the brain. So be sure to perform a steady and thorough warm-up at the start of your workout (see page 18). You will also feel light-headed if your blood glucose levels are too low. It may well be a long time between your lunch and your workout, so have a small snack in the 2 hours before you start. You will find ideas in the snack section on page 218. While you may feel you need a chocolate fix to help you boost your energy levels, avoid this in the 30-minute time gap before you start your workout, as it has been shown to reduce blood sugar levels even further. Instead, try to reach for more easily digestible carbohydrates such as bananas and a few pieces of dried fruit.

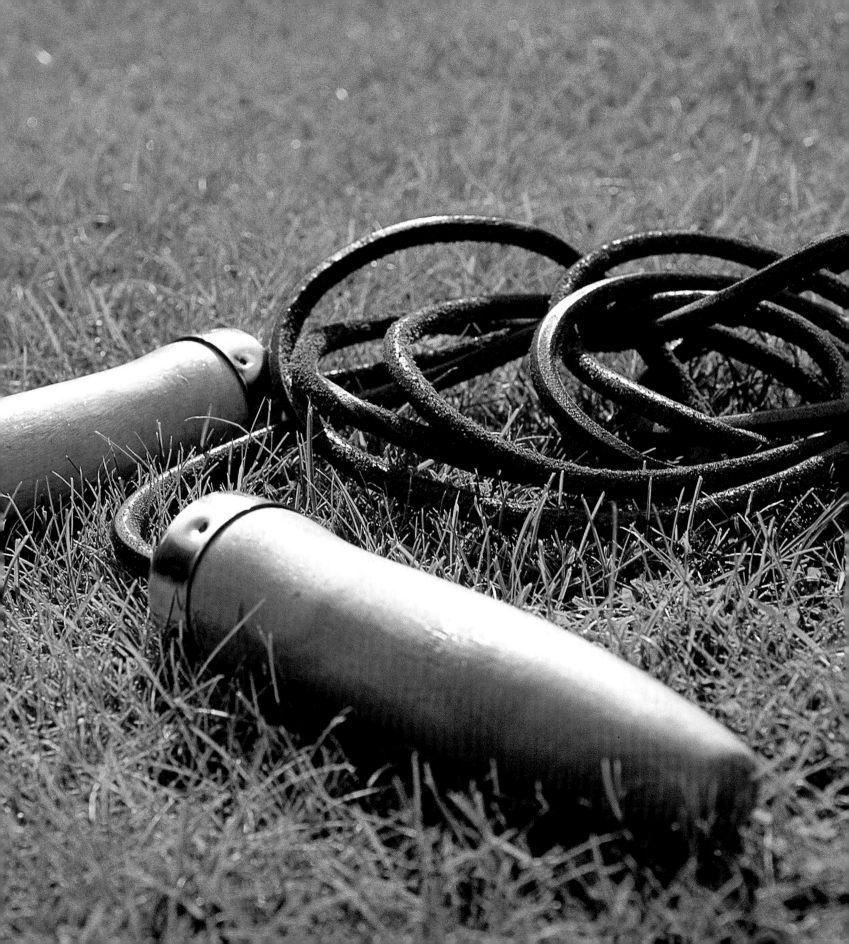

useful information

This is your quick reference section. You'll find user friendly food and exercise tables, tips on what to look for when buying exercise clothing and shoes and a sample studio timeatable to get you moving. Plus there is an activity plan for work and play to keep you motivated all year round. If travelling abroad, check out the glamorous gym locations where you can enjoy the sensation of an aqua massage, or train with views of the most beautiful, scenic and natural workout locations which are completely free to all.

The human body

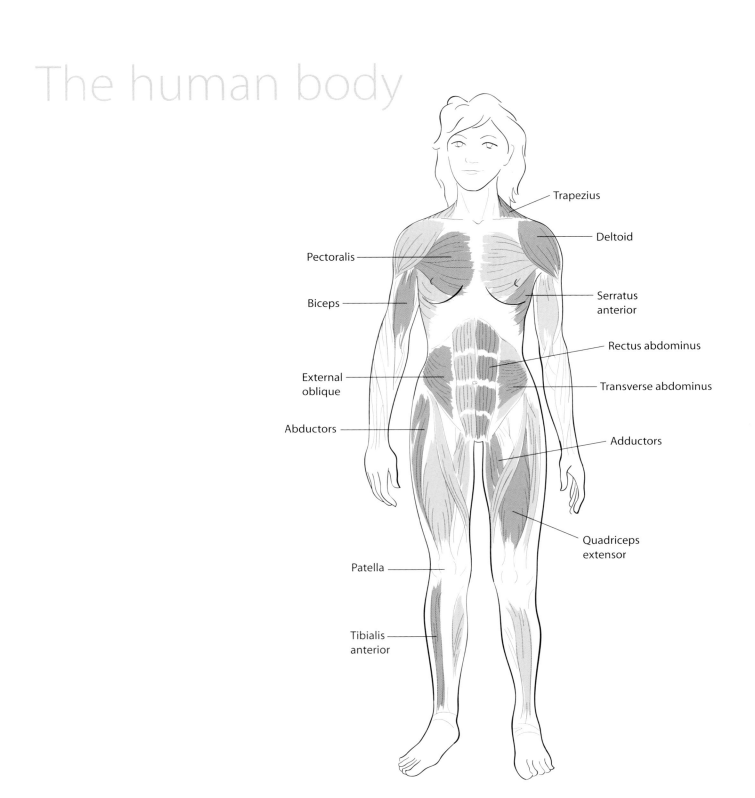

Trapezius

Deltoid

Pectoralis

Serratus anterior

Biceps

Rectus abdominus

External oblique

Transverse abdominus

Abductors

Adductors

Quadriceps extensor

Patella

Tibialis anterior

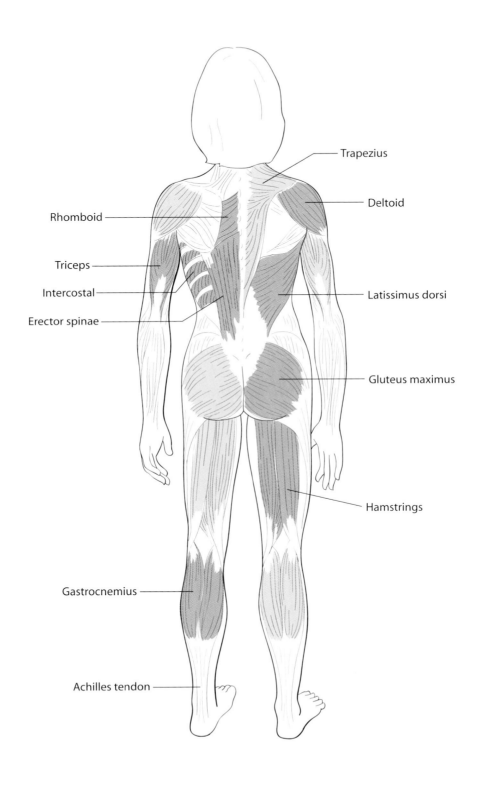

Trapezius

Deltoid

Rhomboid

Triceps

Intercostal

Erector spinae

Latissimus dorsi

Gluteus maximus

Hamstrings

Gastrocnemius

Achilles tendon

Clothing

You may be prepared to pay top money to look great as you do your workout, but does that mean you are going to get a great workout? There is a vast array of sports shoes and clothes now on the market, but whatever you choose there are some fundamental items you need to get right first to ensure you have a comfortable and enjoyable time.

Footwear

This is probably the most important piece of your kit. The issue is not really how much you pay for your shoes, but rather how well they fit your foot and your particular foot strike.

If you are recreational exerciser, you do not need to go out and get the most expensive shoes, nor do you have to have a pair of training shoes for every activity you do. But if you are a serious athlete and focus on performance, it is worth investing in a technical shoe that will offer you the support, protection and features you need.

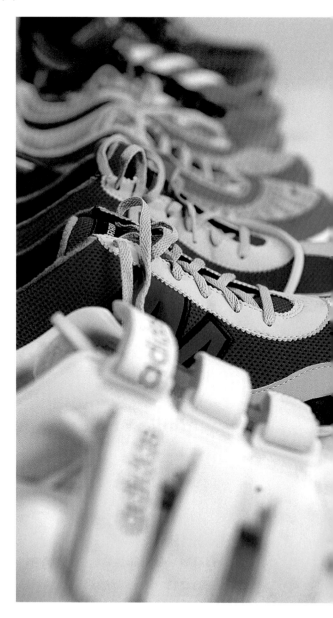

ACTIVITY	WHAT TO LOOK FOR	WHY
Running	Good cushioning in the heel counter and forefoot. The running impact throws the foot forward, so buy a shoe a size bigger than your normal pair of shoes.	Good stability and support in the heel counter is necessary to avoid over-pronation at the ankle. This is particularly important for women, whose feet are more likely to roll in.
Walking	Lightweight breatheable shoe that provides support in the heel counter and forefoot.	Walkers often lead with a 'heel–ball–toe' action as they stride. Heel counter support prevents pronation.
Tennis and racket sports	A sole offering traction on a variety of surfaces, together with support around the forefoot and ankle.	Good lateral support is necessary for side-to-side movements across court. Good traction will prevent sliding on different court surfaces.
Cross-training gym workouts and running activities	A blend of cushioning and stability, with shock absorption in the heel and forefoot. Strong, durable outer sole.	Good cushioning will reduce the impact felt through the forefoot and the heel. A durable outer sole will prolong the life of the trainer that is used for both for outside and indoor workouts.
Aerobics	Good breathing ability, with flexion at the forefoot and a durable sole with good traction. Shoes may be cut low or 'mid' to provide additional support to the ankle.	Aerobic dance routines require a lot of movement in the forefoot, so a shoe with good flexibility in the forefoot will provide ease of movement while offering support to prevent pronation. A traction sole is needed to prevent sliding on dance studio floors.

Sports bra

A good supportive bra is essential as the breast tissue has no muscle and the fatty tissue is supported only by a threadlike mesh of ligaments. Ligaments do not have strong elastic qualities, so it is important to provide support for the breast tissue to avoid over-stretching. Sports bras can be either an inner style worn under your workout clothes or outer style worn as part of your exercise clothing. Look for high-wicking fabrics, which offer ventilation and directional support. Be aware that some inner-style bras have back clasps, which may be a source of discomfort when doing floor exercises.

Outer-style sports bras tend to compress more, and the majority have racing-style backs, so fit discreetly under exercise clothing. Some compression styles work by flattening the breast against the chest wall, creating a less flattering shape, while others provide a natural contour with support panels.

Socks

As you get older you lose the protective fat pads on your feet, so socks can provide protection as well as comfort. Look for pairs that offer durability without bulk and allow your feet to breathe.

Once you have these basics, think about:

- **Long-sleeved T-shirt.** Great for outdoor workouts when the temperature is still cool.
- **Short-sleeved Aertex (or similar) top**. When temperatures warm up, look for materials that allow your skin to breathe, drawing your body's sweat away from your skin.
- **Long trousers.** Look for some sort of stretch material that accommodates your movement.
- **Shorts.** Don't be afraid to get your pins out! Lycra shorts can provide a lot of stretch and freedom of movement as you exercise.
- **Waterproof jacket.** Lightweight shower jackets are useful for rainy days. Choose one that's going to keep you really dry.
- **Hat.** A baseball-style cap can keep your hair out of your eyes and the sun off your face and head.
- **Sunglasses.** Avoid squinting in the sun with sports glasses. Wrap-around styles prevent the glasses falling off and also provide protection at the side of the eyes.

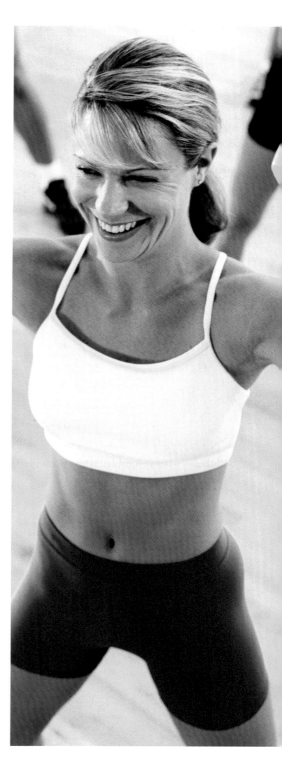

Sample Studio Timetable

TIME	MONDAY	TUESDAY	WEDNESDAY	THURSDAY	FRIDAY
7.00–7.55am	Dawn Yoga	Sunrise Strength Spin	Power Yoga	Mat Pilates	Spin Express
8.00–8.45/9am	Race Day Spin Express Spinning	Ultimate Body Sculpt	Tri Class	Cardio Blast Step Aerobics	Cardio Step Party
9.15–10.15am	Tri Class	Weight Management Course	Mat Pilates	Hatha Yoga	Mat Pilates
10.15–11.15am	Ballet Stretch Works	Fluid Yoga	Total Body Works	Tone Zone	Swiss Ball Toning
11.30am–12.30pm	First Steps to Fitness Course	Project Prime	Hot Stretch and Abs	Project Prime	Total Body Works
12.30–1.30pm	Yoga	Lunchtime Special (aerobics, step or spin)	Dynamic Yoga	Lunchtime Special (aerobics, step or spin)	Bone-up Course
3.30–4.00pm	Tiny Tots' Toning	Yoga Bugs	Brain Gym	Yoga Bugs	Brain Gym
4.30–5.15pm	Teen Time	Yoga Youth	Teen Time	Sports Spot	Capoeira
6.45–7.30 pm	Sculpt and Tone	Tri Workout	Spin Circuits	Sculpt and Tone	Astanga Yoga
7.30–8.30pm	Spin Circuits	Mat Pilates	Yoga	Muscle Sculpt Mania	Hot Stretch and Tone
8.30–9.30pm	Ski Fitness	Capoeira	Hot Stretch and Tone	T'ai Chi	Swiss Ball Toning
9.30–10.30pm	Hydro Fit	Deep Water Running Circuits	General Aquaerobics	Aqua Cardio Circuits	Deep Water Running Circuits

SATURDAY	SUNDAY
Cardio Fat Burner	
Sculpt and Tone	Stretch and Tone
Mat Pilates	Dynamic Yoga
Swiss Ball Toning	Capoeira
Speciality Masterclass Series	Speciality Masterclass Series
T'ai Chi	Spin Express
Spin Circuits	Salsa
	Mat Pilates

The Classes

Cardio/calorie-burning workouts

These workouts entail a minimum of 30 minutes' cardiovascular activity. The remaining section of the class could be designed for either body toning and/or improving mobility and flexibility.

Sample classes: Capoeira, Deep-water Running Circuits, General Aquaerobics, all Spinning Classes. Salsa, Tri Workout, Lunchtime Special, Cardio Fat Burner, Cardio Blast, Cardio Step Party.

Who should attend: Those wanting to lose weight, maintain their weight and body fat levels, improve overall aerobic fitness.

Body-shaping workouts

Classes that aim to tone and shape the body, targeting both upper- and lower-body muscle groups using own body weight, hand weights, tubing and body bars.

Sample classes: Total Body Works, Ultimate Body Sculpt, Hot Stretch and Tone, Swiss Ball Toning, Sculpt and Tone

Who should attend: Those wanting to improve the shape of particular body parts. People who are new to the studio environment may find this an accessible first-time class

Combo workouts

These classes contain both cardiovascular and muscular toning work. Class content is predominantly interval- or circuit-based, with minimum choreography.

Sample classes: Spin Circuits, Ski Fitness, Aqua Cardio Circuits.

Who should attend: Those wanting a total body workout, who prefer unchoreographed workouts and who want to get fit in minimum time.

Mobility and flexibility classes

These classes focus on improving flexibility and mobility, and place a strong emphasis on combining mind-body work to improve overall co-ordination and relaxation. The class content can also be designed to provide muscle-conditioning benefits.

Sample classes: Dawn Yoga, Power Yoga, Dynamic Yoga, Hatha Yoga, Mat Pilates, Stretch and Tone, Fluid Yoga.

Who should attend: Individuals wanting to complement their existing training and improve posture and muscular imbalances.

Healthy youth programmes

These classes are designed to help young people develop cardiovascular fitness, co-ordination, physical self-confidence and balance, within a fun setting.

Sample classes: Tiny Tots (ages 2–4), Sport Spot (ages 13–15), Yoga Bugs (ages 3–8), Brain Gym (ages 4–8).

Specialty masterclass series

Many gyms hold speciality masterclasses at weekends, featuring guest presenters, fitness seminars and innovative classes.

12-month Activity Plan

January may be the month we naturally start out with good intentions, but don't worry if they've disappeared by February; you can pick up this plan any time of the year – just start it from Month 1.

JANUARY (MONTH 1)

Goal: Get the basics right.

This is foundation-building month. So even though you may start the year wanting to blitz your lethargy, forcing yourself to be too energetic all at once is not the answer. You'll risk injury and be more likely to spend the next few months feeling de-motivated, burnt out and maybe even nursing an injury. Focus on increasing your body awareness and improving your stability and posture. Incorporate base-line physical activity into your daily routine, so that when life gets frantic, you have your daily physical activity to fall back on.

What you do: Commit yourself to the Mobility, Posture, Stability and Balance workouts 4 times a week (see pages 99–103 and 126), and a 15-minute cardio workout 3 times a week (see Cardiovascular chapter, pages 34–63). Walk a minimum of 4,000 steps every day.

Top Tip: Skip fad diets – they will only decrease your metabolism.

FEBRUARY (MONTH 2)

Goal: Rev-up your metabolism.

Boost your lean muscle mass and you'll give your metabolic rate a kick-start. It will help you develop whole-body toning and strengthen your body as you raise your activity levels. By the end of the month you'll expend more calories every minute, even when you are not exercising.

What you do: Commit yourself to resistance training. Add the Workout in a Suitcase (see page 184) or Wall Workout (see page 178) to your programme twice a week.

Introduce abdominal Best Body Bits exercises (see page 67) to build a strong torso and core stability.

Top Tip: Eat breakfast – eating something in the morning has been shown to boost metabolism by 30%, and curb mid-morning snacking. Don't forget to overload your muscles! (See page 62 for details)

MARCH (MONTH 3)

Goal: Beat exercise boredom.

You are 8 weeks in, and it is now that your motivation may start to wane. Make a list of the real reasons why you want to improve your health to keep you focused (see page 157 for more motivation tips).

What you do: Pick a fun race event for a few a months time to work towards.

Keep a training log (see page 158).

Introduce a Playtime Workout to your programme (see page 196) and do it with a friend.

Top Tip: Glam-up your training. Select a race event that will be a big enough challenge for you to have to work towards it. Go for some exciting location event (such as the Paris to Versailles 16km race, or the Prague Half Marathon) to make a weekend of it.

Don't forget your Stability Workout (page 126). It will lessen the risk of injury as you increase your training.

APRIL (MONTH 4)

Goal: Time to step up a gear. By now you have created a strong foundation in your posture and base fitness and now is the time to build on that.

What you do: Increase daily walking targets to 7,000 steps.

Hit the outdoors with the Cardio Calorie Blast walking programme (see page 48). If you are a jogger, increase the pace to suit you.

Introduce beginner yoga postures after your cardio calorie burn to reduce muscle shortening and compensate for any misalignment when you walk.

Top Tip: Fortify your diet with antioxidants to boost your immune system. If you are taking a supplement, check that it contains selenium to boost feel-good brain activity.

MAY (MONTH 5)

Goal: Burn that body fat.

Time to streamline you body and realize healthy body fat levels with increased cardiovascular work.

What you do: Build up your daily walking targets to between 7,000 and 10,000 steps (see page 37).

Introduce interval training into your cardio programme. If you are preparing for a race event, up your speed training (see page 58).

Top Tip: Start body-brushing to stimulate circulation and improve skin texture.

JUNE (MONTH 6)

Goal: Build body confidence.

Focus on building your physical self esteem.

What you do: Commit to your abdominal Best body Bits workout (see page 77) 4 times a week. If you are thinking about going on holiday this month, don't forget you've still got time to start your Build a Beach Body Plan (see page 198). The compound exercises will deliver results fast.

Top Tip: Reduce Posture and Mobility Workouts (page 99-103) to twice a week, but pick out key moves to incorporate into other workouts.

JULY (MONTH 7)

Goal: Downsize your workouts.

Now is the month to be more creative with your time. Reduce your personal structured exercise programme and instead, get outdoors. Inspire and involve the whole family to be more active.

What you do: Resolve to walk your 10,000 steps daily. Introduce your Water Workout (see page 49).

Get the kids to try their Yoga Bug postures (page 140). Plan activity adventures – hike to a national park, or picnic at down on a beach.

Top Tips: Schedule in technology-free time-zones at weekends and give the family the task of choosing their activity for each weekend.

AUGUST (MONTH 8)

Goal: Change your exercise environment. Take the opportunity to step outside your regular exercise zone and explore different locations and mediums.

What you do: Mix things up this month – if you are a runner take your activity to water with deep-water running. If you tend to exercise outside, explore indoor activities, such as your local club's studio timetable. Or put your mind and body to the test with rock climbing.

Top Tips: Consider investing in new exercise shoes; they may look good from the outside but if you have put 500 miles plus through them, it's time to get a new pair.

SEPTEMBER (MONTH 9)

Goal: Move more often.

Focus on accumulating more daily physical activity. If you are preparing for next month's race event, you can afford to ease off on your training so that you are ready to peak when the time comes.

What you do: Record an activity audit detailing how much you move daily.

Introduce your Car Workout (see page 182). The changing seasons may mean you will be spending more time in the car.

Schedule moving times into your day. Aim to get out and move at least 3 times each day.

Top Tips: Move your body for 10 minutes before you open your purse each day! Think of something you buy on a daily basis and make a commitment to walk before you spend any money.

OCTOBER (MONTH 10)

Goal: Your race event.

This is the month you have been working towards. Ease off your training a couple of weeks before the event, and boost your flexibility work to prepare your muscles.

What you do: Add a Yoga Workout (see page 113) to your programme 3 times a week.

Introduce a Stability Workout (see page 126) to ensure muscle balance.

Practise drinking on the move in the last few runs you do. You will need to master the skill of collecting your drinks from the water stations on the course.

Top Tips: Remember the event is your victory lap for all your hard training. Enjoy it!

NOVEMBER (MONTH 11)

Goal: Exercise vacation.

Take it easy this month. You have achieved your goals and your body deserves a rest. Focus on restoring the body and building balance back into your programme.

What you do: Introduce a group mind-body class such as t'ai chi or yoga. Complement this with the T'ai Chi Workout on page 105.

Restore your body with the One-Hit Wonder postures on page 171.

Don't neglect your daily minimum walking targets.

Top Tips: Book a massage or body treatment. Spoil yourself!

DECEMBER (MONTH 12)

Goal: Exercise time management.

The seasonal festivities can be quite hectic. With so much to plan, make sure you schedule in your 'me' time. Make sure your exercise does not get shoved to the bottom of the 'To Do' list, never to get done.

What you do: Learn how to get quality sleep with the 'Quiet Eyes' exercise and the Relaxation Meditation (see pages 169 and 170).

Add variety to your programme with the Wall Workout (see page 178). This workout will deliver results fast.

Get outside at weekends with the winter playtime workout.

Top Tips: Enjoy the festivities and don't beat yourself up if you are not as active as usual or indulge in too much seasonal fare. It is important to enjoy yourself, your family and your life. Happy Holidays!

Your Calorie Store Cupboard

In this chart you will find the calorie and fat content of a variety of popular foods. The exact nutrient content varies between brands, so remember it is always useful to have a look at the food labels when you are shopping. As a useful exercise try to assess your calorie intake for several days and then divide by the number of days you record – this will provide you with a more realistic reflection of your daily calorie intake. It is important to eat a variety of different foodstuffs, so cast your eye over the list to check you are having a range of foods, especially from the fruit and vegetables. If you are used to kilojoules, simply multiply the calory value by 4.2.

FOOD	PORTION	FAT (GRAMS)	CALORIES	FOOD	PORTION	FAT (GRAMS)	CALORIES
CARBOHYDRATE SOURCES				Cabbage	100g/4oz	0.5	25
Fruit				Carrots	1 medium	0.1	26
Apple	1 medium	0.5	82	Courgettes	100g/4oz	0.4	18
Apricot	1	0.1	16	Cucumber	1 medium	0.3	24
Avocado	1 no skin, no stone	30	306	Green beans	100g/4oz	0.1	31
Banana	medium	0.5	108	Lettuce	100g/4oz	0.1	12
Blackberries	100g/4oz	0.3	52	Mange tout	100g/4oz	0.2	32
Blueberries	100g/4oz	0.3	56	Mushrooms	100g/4oz	0.3	25
Grapefruit	1/2 fruit	0.1	53	Onions	1 large	0.2	57
Grapes	100g/4oz	0.6	71	Peas	100g/4oz	0.4	81
Honeydew melon	1 wedge 1/8 of melon	0.1	43	Pumpkin	100g/4oz	0.1	26
Kiwi	1 medium no skin	0.3	46	Spinach	100g/4oz	0.3	22
Lemon	1	0.2	17	Sweet Corn	1 cob	1.1	77
Lime	1	0.1	20	Turnip	100g/4oz	0.1	27
Nectarine	1	0.6	67	**Starches**			
Mango	1 no skin no stone	0.5	134	Bagel	1 large	1.5	195
Olives	1	0.4	5	Bread, fruit	1 slice	1.1	71
Orange	1 medium	0.1	62	Bread, pitta	1 large	0.7	165
Peach	1 medium	0.0	42	Bread, white	1 slice	0.9	66
Pear	1 medium	0.6	98	Bread, wholegrain	1 slice	0.8	73
Pineapple	1 thick slice	0.3	41	Breakfast cereal, bran flake	100g/4oz	2.2	320
Raspberries	100g/4oz	0.5	49	Breakfast cereal, puffed rice	100g/4oz	0.4	396
Strawberries	1	0	5	Breakfast cereal, Muesli	100g/4oz	6.0	364
Watermelon	1 wedge 1/16 of melon	1.2	92	Chips	100g/4oz	6	160
Vegetables				Pasta	100g/4oz	1.5	371
Artichoke	1 medium	0.2	60	Porridge oats	100g/4oz	7.0	389
Asparagus	100g/4oz	0.2	23	Potato, mashed with butter & milk	100g/4oz	4.0	110
Broccoli	1 stalk	0.5	42	Potato, jacket	1 medium	0.2	220

FOOD	PORTION	(FAT GRAMS)	CALORIES
Rice, brown	100g	2.9	370
Rice, white	100g	0.5	370
PROTEIN			
Almonds	100g/4oz	50	578
Bacon, fat trimmed	100g/4oz	7	136
Baked beans in tomato sauce	100g/4oz	0.4	93
Beef	100g/4oz	10	218
Brazil nuts	100g/4oz	66	656
Chicken	100g/4oz	4	165
Chick peas	100g/4oz	1.1	119
Cod	100g/4oz	0.6	82
Egg	1 large	5	74
Haddock, smoked	100g/4oz	0.9	116
Ham, all visible fat cut off	100g/4oz	6.0	127
Hamburger	100g/4oz	30	342
Kidneys	100g/4oz	3	99
Kidney beans, tinned	100g/4oz	0.5	127
Lamb	100g/4oz	7	144
Liver	100g/4oz	5	139
Peanut butter	100g/4oz	49	589
Peanuts, dry-roasted	100g/4oz	51	594
Pork lean only	100g/4oz	10	212
Prawns	100g/4oz	0.4	69
Salmon fillet	100g/4oz	6.0	142
Salmon, tinned in brine, drained	100g/4oz	6.0	139
Salmon, smoked	100g/4oz	4	117
Sardines, tinned in olive oil, drained	100g/4oz	11.3	195
Sausages	100g/4oz	40	417
Trout	100g/4oz	4	104
Turkey	100g/4oz	0.7	111
Tuna steak	100g/4oz	5.0	144
Tuna, tinned in oil, drained	100g/4oz	8	198
Walnuts	100g/4oz	65	654

FOOD	PORTION	FAT (GRAMS)	CALORIES
MILK AND DAIRY SOURCES			
Cottage cheese	100g/4oz	2.9	95
Cheddar cheese	100g/4oz	33	402
Cream cheese	100g/4oz	35	349
Brie cheese	100g/4oz	27	333
Edam cheese	100g/4oz	27	356
Goats' cheese	100g/4oz	30	364
Parmesan cheese	100g/4oz	30	455
Cream, double, reduced fat	100g/4oz	36	349
Milk, full-fat	100ml/4fl oz	3.3	61
Milk, semi-skimmed	100ml/4fl oz	1.7	49
Milk, skimmed	100ml/4fl oz	0.1	35
Yoghurt, natural low fat	100g/4oz	1.5	63
Yoghurt, fruit low fat	100g/4oz	1.5	99
Sour cream	100g/4oz	20	214
FATS AND SUGARS			
Butter	100g/4oz	81	717
Chocolate	50g bar	15	255
Chocolate biscuits	100g/4oz	15	453
Chocolate éclair	1 large	15	262
Cream cake	1 large	17	238
Ice cream	100g/4oz	11	216
Lard	100g/4oz	100	902
Margarine, reduced fat	100g/4oz	38	345
Mayonnaise	100g/4oz	33	389
Olive oil	1 tablespoon	14	119
Potato crisps	100g/4oz	32	491

Calorie Expenditure During Activity

This chart shows you the energy expended doing different activities. You'll find values for your daily activities as well as more structured exercise and physical activity. To help you I have listed them as in the different chapters of the book. Each activity is given a calorie value per minute based on a 68kg/10st 7lb individual. Your weight has a direct effect upon the number of calories your body expends to achieve that movement. To personalize the values to you add 10% for every 6.8kg/15lb over 68kg/10st 7lb and subtract 10% for every 16.8kg/15lb under 68kg/10st 7lb . Some activities list a range of calories expended per minute. Remember that the intensity of your movements will also affect the amount of energy your body uses as it moves. Use this chart to help work out your estimated daily energy expenditure.

ACTIVITY	CALORIES/ MINUTE
Cardiovascular exercise	
Canoeing 4–6.4kph/2.5–4.0mph	3.0–7.0
Volleyball – active, recreation, competitive	3.4–8.0
Golfing	4.0
Table tennis	5.0
Rowing – recreational, vigorous	5.0-15
Cycling, 8–24kph/5–15 mph	5.0–12.0
Skating, recreational – vigorous	5-15.0
Tennis	7.0–11.0
Water skiing	8.0
Football, active midfield position	9.0
Skipping	10–15.0
Downhill skiing, moderate to steep incline	8–20.0
Downhill ski Racing	16.5
Cross country skiing 4.8–16kph/3–10 mph	9.0–20.0
Swimming, gently	6.0
Swimming front crawl, 23–46m/25–50yds/min	6.0–12.5
Swimming butterfly, 23–46m/25–50yds/min	14.0
Aqua aerobics	6.0–8.0
Deep-water jogging, vigorously	11.0
Swimming backstroke, 23–46m/25–50yds/min	6.0–12.5
Swimming breaststroke	6.0–12.5
Dancing – salsa, modern, disco	4.2 – 6.0
Line dancing	7.7
Power-walking, 15% incline at 5.6kmp/3.5 mph	11.0–15.0
Walking, 5.6kmp/3.5 mph	5.6–7.0
Running, 12-minute mile (8kph/5 mph)	10.0
Running 8-minute mile (12kpm/7.5 mph)	15.0
Running 6-minute mile (16kmp/10mph)	20.0

ACTIVITY	CALORIES/ MINUTE
Resistance exercise	
Circuit training	6.0 –8.0
Muscular strength training	8.0
Muscular endurance training	4.5–7.0
Flexibility exercise	
Pilates	4.0–6.0
Power yoga	5.0–7.0
Gentle yoga	4.0
Stretching	3.0
T'ai chi	4.0
Lifestyle	
Sleeping	1.2
Lazing in bed	1.3
Sitting at a desk reading	1.3
Chatting	1.5
Standing	1.5
Sitting at a desk writing	2.5
Washing and dressing	2.5
Driving a car	2.8
Walking around your home	3.1
Making the beds	3.5
Ironing clothes	4.2
Gardening – weeding	5.5
Walking downstairs	7.0
Gardening – digging	8.5
Walking upstairs	10.0–18.0

NB. Absolute intensity (METS) values are approximate mean values for men. Mean values for women are approximately 1–2 METS lower than for men.

Carbohydrate-containing foods with a **high** glycaemic index (>85)

The foods in this table are generally regarded as high GI foods, providing a faster release of blood glucose – they are best eaten after endurance exercise to help with muscle fuel replenishment.

FOOD GROUP	FOOD	Serving size (g/ml), giving 50g carbohydrate	Fat per serving (g)
Cereals	White bread	210g	2
	Wholemeal bread	120g	3
	Rye bread (light)	104g	4
	Bagel	89g	2
	Pastry (shortcrust)	90g	29
	Rice (wholegrain)	196g	1
	Rice (white)	169g	0.5
Breakfast cereals	Cornflakes	59g	1
	Muesli	76g	6
	Shredded Wheat	74g	2
	Weetabix	71g	2
Biscuits and confectionery	Digestive biscuits	76g	16
	Crispbread (rye)	71g	1.5
	Plain cracker	66g	8
	Chocolate nougat bar (contains sucrose and glucose)	75g	14
Vegetables	Sweetcorn	219g	5
	Broad beans	704g	4
	Parsnips	370g	Trace
	Potato (instant)	310g	0.5
	Potato (boiled)	254g	Trace
	Potato (baked)	200g	Trace
Fruit	Raisins	78g	Trace
	Banana	260g	1
Sugars	Glucose	50g	0
	Maltose	50g	0
	Honey	67g	(wax only) 3
	Sucrose	50g	0
	Molasses	113ml	0
	Corn syrup	63g	0
Beverages	6% sucrose solution	833ml	0

FOOD GROUP	FOOD	Serving size (g/ml), giving 50g carbohydrate	Fat per serving (g)
	7.5% maltodextrin and sugar	666ml	0
	10% corn syrup-carbonated drink	500ml	0
	20% maltodextrin	250ml	0

Carbohydrate-containing foods with a **moderate** glycaemic index (61–84)

Moderate and low GI foods release glucose into the bloodstream more gradually, and therefore make a good breakfast.

FOOD GROUP	FOOD	Serving size (g), giving 50g carbohydrate	Fat per serving (g)
Cereals	Spaghetti/macaroni	198	1
	Noodles (oriental)	370	14
Breakfast cereals	Wheatbran nuggets	232	13
	Porridge (oatmeal)	69	1
Biscuits and confectionery	Oatmeal biscuits	79	15
	Rich tea biscuits	67	11
	Sponge cake	93	6
Vegetables	Potato (sweet)	249	1
	Yam	168	trace
	Potato chips	100	40
Fruit	Grapes (black)	323	trace
	Grapes (green)	310	trace
	Orange	420–600	trace

Carbohydrate-containing foods with a **low** glycaemic index (<60)

FOOD GROUP	FOOD	Serving size (g/ml), giving 50g carbohydrate	Fat per serving (g)
Fruit	Apples	400g	trace
	Apple sauce	290g	trace
	Cherries	420g	trace
	Dates (dried)	78g	trace
	Figs (raw)	526g	trace
	Grapefruit (canned)	300g	trace
	Peaches	450–500g	trace
	Plums	500–550g	trace
Legumes	Butter beans	292g	1
	Baked beans	485g	2
	Haricot beans	301g	2
	Chick peas	305g	5
	Red lentils	294g	2
Sugars	Fructose	50g	0
Dairy products	Ice cream	202g	13
	Milk (full-fat)	1.1 litres	40
	Milk (semi-skim)	1.0 litres	1
	Yoghurt (plain, low-fat)	800g	8
	Yoghurt (fruit, low-fat)	280g	3
Soup	Tomato soup	734ml	6

Vitamins and minerals

Vitamin/Mineral	RDA	UL	Food sources
Calcium	Ages 19–50: 1,000mg Over 50: 1,200mg	2,500mg	Dairy foods, dark green leafy vegetables, legumes, fortified foods
Magnesium	Women: 320mg; men: 420mg	350mg*	Nuts, legumes, whole grains, soya beans, seafood, drak-green leafy vegetables
Phosphorus	700mg	Ages 19–70: 4,000mg; Over 70: 3,000mg	Animal products such as meat, fish, poultry, eggs, dairy products; processed and prepared foods; soft drinks.
Vitamin D	Ages 19–50: 200 IU. 51–70 400 IU; over 70 600 IU	2,000 IU	Oily fish and fish oils, egg yolks, butter, vitamin D-fortified milk
Fluoride	Women: 3mg; men: 4 mg	10mg	Water, fortified systems (fluoride found naturally or fortified) dental products
Folate	400mcg	1,000mcg*	Dark green leafy vegetables, beans, orange juice, cantaloupe melon, sweet potatoes, foods made with wholegrain or enriched flour.
Niacin	Women: 14mg; men: 16mg	35mg	Protein-rich foods such as meat, peanuts, poultry, legumes, milk and eggs
Vitamin B6	Ages 19–50: 1.3 mg, women over 50: 1.5 mg; men over 50 1.7mg	100mg	Offal, poultry, fish, egg yolk, legumes, peanuts, walnuts
Choline	(Adequate intake) women: 425mg; men: 550mg	3,500mg	Legumes, red meat, milk, wholegrain cereals, egg yolk
Vitamin C	Women: 75mg; men: 90mg. (Smokers: add 35mg.)	2,000mg	Vegetables and fruits such as citrus fruits, tomatoes, dark green leafy vegetables and potatoes
Vitamin E	15mg	1,000mg *	Nuts, seeds and their oils, vegetable oils, green leafy vegetables.
Selenium	55mcg	400mcg	Seafood, liver, meat, milk, eggs, grains
Vitamin A	Women: 700mcg; men: 900mcg	3,000mcg	Liver, oily fish, fortified foods (milk, breakfast cereals)
Copper	900mcg	10mg	Wholegrain breads and cereals, seafood, nuts, eggs, poultry, legumes, dark green leafy vegetables
Iodine	150 mcg	1.1mg	Iodized salt, plants, seafood
Iron	Women ages 19–50: 18mg, women over 50: 8mg; men: 8mg	45mg	Red meat, dried fruits, legumes, dark green leafy vegetables, wholegrain or enriched grain products
Manganese	(Adequate intake) Women: 1.8mg; men: 2.3mg	11mg	Green leafy vegetables, meats, tea, wholegrain breads, cereals, legumes, nuts
Molybdenum	45mcg	2mg	Whole grains, breads, cereals, legumes, leafy vegetables and nuts
Zinc	Women: 8mg; men: 11mg	40mg	Red meat, seafood, milk, egg yolk, wholegrain breads and cereals, fortified foods

* From supplements and fortified foods only. The nutrients that occur naturally in food are not included in this value.

Function	When too much is not a good thing
Builds strong bones and teeth; is vital for nerve transmission, muscle contraction, blood clotting	Kidney damage, kidney stones; blocks absorption of other nutrients (iron and zinc)
Is a major bone constituent and is instrumental in enzyme systems, protein synthesis, nerve transmission, muscle contraction.	Diarrhoea, nausea, abdominal cramping
Is a structural part of cells; contributes to bone and soft tissue growth.	Damage to kidneys and bones
Regulates calcium absorption and deposits into bone.	Elevated blood calcium levels, which may lead to kidney and heart damage.
Reduces tooth decay.	Discoloration of teeth and bone problems
Contributes to protein metabolism and production of neurotransmitters.	Can mask or lead to a vitamin B12 deficiency, potentially causing irreversible nerve damage.
Contributes to carbohydrate metabolism and red blood cell formation.	Skin flushing, nausea, vomiting, potential liver damage.
Contributes to protein, carbohydrate, fat and cholesterol metabolism; haemoglobin production; and the proper functioning and growth of the red blood cells.	Potential irreversible nerve damage, difficulty walking
Contributes to fat and cholesterol metabolism and the manufacture of neurotransmitters, reduces or prevents fatty liver.	Fishy body and breath odour, sweating, salivation, liver problems, decreased blood pressure
Provides antioxidant benefits; plays major role in collagen formation	Diarrhoea, kidney stones
Provides antioxidant benefits; acts as an anticoagulant.	Haemorrhaging
Provides antioxidant benefits.	Hair loss, nail damage
Essential for eyesight, immune function, gene expression, reproduction, growth and good skin.	Irreversible liver damage, birth defects
Helps develop nerves, bone, blood and connective tissue.	Liver damage
Helps produce thyroid hormones.	Thyroid problems
Shuttles the oxygen in the bloodstream; contributes to collagen synthesis and immune function; prevents anaemia.	Gastro-intestinal upset, potential increased risk of heart disease and cancer.
Contributes to bone formation and protein, carbohydrate and fat metabolism.	Central nervous system problems
Plays important role in enzyme systems and iron metabolism.	Reproductive and growth problems
Contributes to enzyme and insulin activity, protein synthesis, bone structure, gene expression and immune system function.	Suppression of immune response, decrease in HDL cholesterol, blocking of copper absorption.

Glamorous Gym Locations

Berlin

Oasis Fitness Gesundheitszentrum

When packing your suitcase don't forget your *Badenhosen*, as the highlight of this club is the Olympic-sized pool. If you really want to know what it feels like to swim 100m in Olympic time, here is your chance! If swimming is not your thing, break sweat in the well-equipped gym or with less effort in one of the 3 saunas. As it's open till 10pm, there really is no excuse for being a couch potato once you've finished that business report!

Stresemannstrabe, 74 Kreuzberg, Berlin, Germany

Tel: (+49) 262 6661

Brussels

Champneys

The one thing you just must do at this club is to have the aqua massage. You don't even have to get wet: you just lie down fully clothed as you enjoy the sensation of water jets pummelling your body through super-dry plastic covering. And if that is not enough to leave you feeling refreshed, there's piped music in the relaxation rooms, and plunge pools and therapies to try out before you sweat away your day in the state-of-the-art gym. If you are a regular European traveller and a member of Champneys in Europe, you can enjoy the Champneys hospitality free of charge in London too.

Champneys Brussels, Avenue Louise 71B,

1050 Brussels, Belgium

Tel: (+32) 02 542 46 66

London

The Third Space

Kitted out with the latest top-of-the-range fitness equipment, this £13 million health temple is the darling of the media fraternity in London's trendy Soho area. The runners and bikers have their own personal MP3 players and are netted up to surf, e-mail and watch mpegs as they pound the flesh. A 75m/245ft climbing wall may prove a challenge for some, or you can go several rounds with your own military trainer in the competition-sized boxing ring. If you don't fancy that, you can always get some serious run-training in the high-altitude run chamber. And the 20m/65ft pool is treated with ozone, not chlorine, so you won't get sore eyes!

13 Sherwood Street, London W1

Tel: (+44) 020 7439 6333

Milan

Club 10 Health and Beauty

This laid-back club is more the place to be seen than the place to break sweat. Located in one of Milan's grandest hotels, the beautiful setting boasts a well-equipped gym for beautiful people. Supermodels mostly prefer to swim a few laps of the bijou swimming pool or pummel their stress away in the whirlpool before indulging in the sauna, steam and beauty rooms for treatments.

Hotel Principe di Savoia, Milan, Italy

Tel: (+39) 02 62301

New York

Chelsea Piers Complex

Your family will need a week rather than day to enjoy the extensive all-lifestyle facilities at the Pier. The Sports Club at Pier 60 is renowned as the best gym in the world, and for good reason. Why not practise your running technique on the 3km/1.8 mile indoor running track while taking in the breathtaking views across the Hudson River? With two exercise studios (boasting over 150 classes a week, ranging from 'urban yoga' to 'warrior girl workouts'), a Pilates machine studio, boxing ring, volleyball courts, and a huge pool, you will be quite ready to lounge on the sundeck before going off to ice skate, rock climb, go-kart... Better still, head for a relaxation treatment at the Origins Spa located inside.

Pier 60 at 23rd Street at the West Side Highway,

New York City, USA

Tel: (+1) 212 336 6262

Sao Paolo

Centro De Practicas Esportivas de Universidade de Sao Paolo

If you go for a workout here, you may leave bemoaning the fact that facilities like these were unimaginable when you were at school! This phenomenal university illustrates the fact that not all campuses are created equal. This one can boast a multi-purpose gym, an aqua park including an Olympic-sized pool, tennis courts, a 4km/2.5 mile cycling track around the campus and a chess room to get a brain workout as well as a brawn workout!

Praca 02, Prof. Rubiao Meira 61, Cidade

Universitaria, Sao Paolo, Brazil

Tel: (+11) 3818 3565/3361

Tokyo

Club on the Park

If the price of membership does not give you a head rush, the altitude will. Located on the 47th floor of the Park Hyatt Hotel, this boasts a view of Mount Fuji on a clear day. When you are done with the myriad

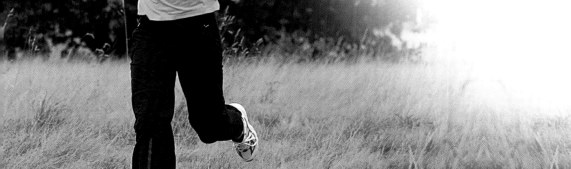

machines, equipment and workout gizmos, enjoy 360° body showers. And it really would be a shame to go all that way and not enjoy some ancient Oriental body treatments: reflexology or Shiatsu can be great to relieve that jet-lag.

Park Hyatt, 3-7-1-2 Nishi-Shinjuku, Shinjuku – ku, Tokyo, Japan

Tel: (+81) 3 5322 1234

Try some of these unforgettable jogging routes for an invigorating cardio blast.

Dominica

On the rainforest trail in Dominica's Northern Forest Reserve, through a parrot sanctuary, and up to the top of the island's highest mountain.

London

Run east along the south bank of the Thames starting at Westminster Bridge and you will take in the famous sites – the Houses of Parliament, St Paul's Cathedral, the Tate Modern and Tower Bridge. Feeling fit? Run over Tower Bridge and back along the north embankment.

Minneapolis

Marvel at the beauty of the 'Chain of Lakes': the Lake of the Isles, Lake Calhoun and Lake Harriet.

Prague

To take in the cultural views of Old Prague, start in Kampa park, run over Charles Bridge and up to the home of Charles (name to confirm). The hills can be pretty challenging as you stride past the wall that kept the poor out of the royal vista. Remember, power-walking can be great for your gluteals, so don't panic if you need to walk.

Rio de Janeiro

The route may be down hill but you need to be pretty fit to run all the way down to Copacabana beach. The running route through the national park is stunningly beautiful, so you may prefer to hire a mountain bike so that your enjoyment of the scenery is less arduous.

Sydney

Within walking distance of the city, Centennial Park offers a 4km/2.5 mile run against a car-free picturesque backdrop. Or if you fancy a more watery vista, start at Vaucluse and head along the coastal path down into Bondi, run along the beach and continue along the headlands and down into Tamarama. Running back to Vaucluse, you will be distracted on the last few hills, by the the views of Sydney Harbour Bridge and the Opera House.

index

acknowledgements

A big thanks to my clients and friends who modelled and battled with the elements on a cold and slightly damp February day – your support was really appreciated!
Freddy Brunt; Mairi, Andrew, Ross and Max Chapman; Clodagh, Charlie, Sophie, Charlotte and Rupert Curtis; Robyn Gilkes; Delores Lee; Sarah, Isabella and Rupert Stanley; Jilly Visser; Kelly and Judy Wilden.

To young Joshua Stagg who is always happy to be pushed in his pram – and thank you to Mum Sue for letting him commence his modeling career early!

And of course many thanks to Juliet Turner; Becky Riley, who has since given birth to Lucy on May 30th 2002 and Emily Fenwick Klenell.

To Fenella Lindsell for her continual co-operation and support with the use of the Art of Health and Yoga centre and all her yoga bugs (Felix, Lewis, Alyssia, Katie, Jemima and friends) who were just great at practicing their bug moves again and again. A big thank you to all their Mummys too.

To Mark Raudva and his Tai Chi class at the Art of Health and Yoga centre, your calmness is quite contagious.

To Madelaine Backlund and her studio team at Madelaine Backlund Pilates especially Anastasia Theodoridou.

A special thanks to Jane Tyler for styling and makeup and to Fran Yorke, our photographer who handled all weather conditions with a great sense of humour!

Thanks also to Dr. Jules Eaden and Dr. Tim Evans for their medical contributions to the text.

I would also like to thank Richard Branson and his fantastic staff at Virgin Atlantic for their co-operation with filming at their headquarters for the airplane workouts.

Thanks to the following companies:
Viva (UK) Ltd for the loan of the Casall sportswear (www.casall.com   +44 (0)1458 273394).
First Sport for the loan of equipment (www.firstsport.co.uk   +44 (0)191 5182002).
Peter Cox at PCA Creative for the illustrations on pages 234–5 (www.pca-design.co.uk   +44 (0)1531 633033).
LA Fitness for the use of their gym in the Waldorf Hotel, London (www.lafitness.co.uk   +44 (0)7 3668080). See location on pages 47–54, 68–9, 82–5 (top), 88–9, 198–9 (bottom), 200 (middle) and 201 (top).

Many, many thanks to all at Kyle Cathie, especially Kyle, herself, for her unfailing support and Sheila Davies and Sarah Epton for their patience, commitment and dedication.

A final special thanks to all my clients who continue to be a source of inspiration and enjoyment – it is you who motivate me. Thank you.

Activeaction
132–134 Lots Road
London, SW10 0RJ
www.activeaction.com

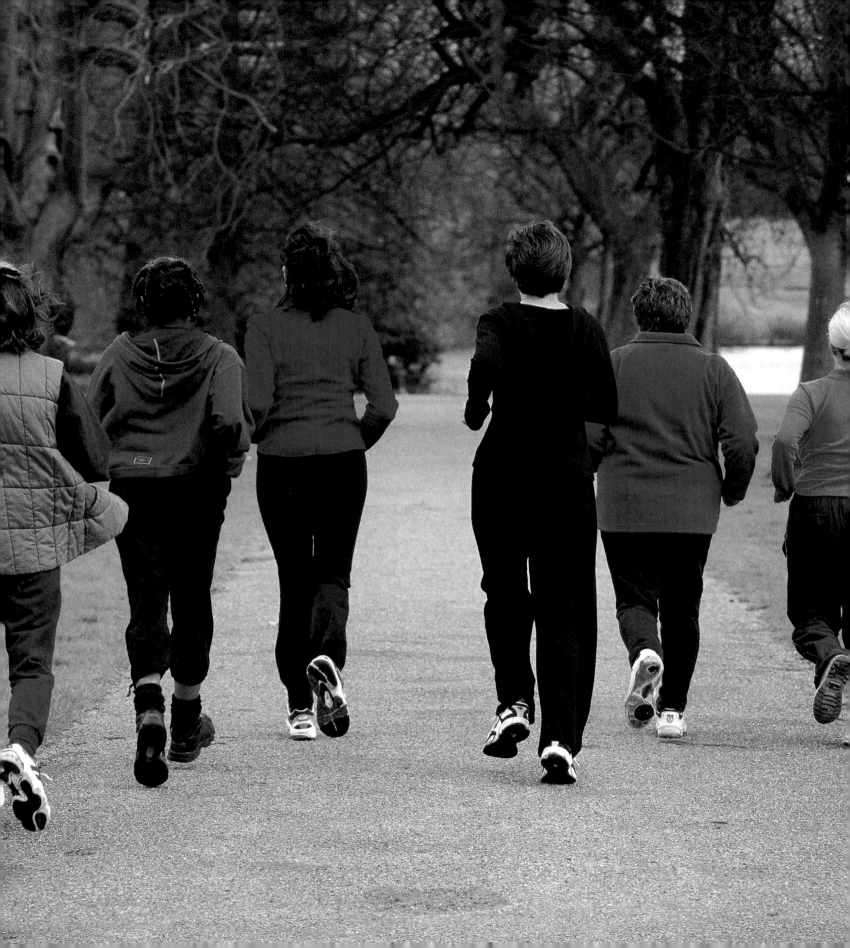